BEYOND CARBS

The Best Simple and Effective pathway to Diabetes Control for a Healthy Life

Robert M. Rowell

INTRODUCTION

DECODING CARBS AND DIABETES

Understanding the Carbohydrate Conundrum in Diabetes

• The Basics of Diabetes

Diabetes, a prevalent metabolic disorder, disrupts the body's ability to regulate blood sugar (glucose) effectively. For individuals navigating this condition, the role of carbohydrates in the diet takes center stage. Carbs, found in various foods, significantly impact blood sugar levels, making them a crucial element to understand for effective diabetes management.

• The Carbohydrate Spectrum: Simple vs. Complex

Carbohydrates come in different forms, broadly categorized as simple and complex. Simple carbohydrates, often referred to as sugars, are found in foods like candies, pastries, and sugary beverages. They are quickly broken down, leading to rapid spikes in blood sugar levels. In contrast, complex carbohydrates, prevalent in whole grains, fruits, and vegetables, consist of longer chains of sugar molecules. The body takes more time to break them down, resulting in a slower and steadier release of glucose.

• Glycemic Index (GI) Unveiled

To navigate the carbohydrate landscape effectively, understanding the Glycemic

Index (GI) becomes paramount. The GI is a numerical scale that ranks carbohydrates based on how quickly they raise blood sugar levels. Foods with a high GI cause a rapid spike, while those with a low GI release glucose more gradually, offering a sustained energy release. This index serves as a valuable tool for making informed food choices in diabetes management.

• The Impact of Carbs on Blood Sugar Levels

Every carbohydrate consumed has a direct impact on blood sugar levels. When we eat, carbohydrates are broken down into glucose, which enters the bloodstream, causing blood sugar levels to rise. For individuals with diabetes, this process can be disrupted, leading to challenges in maintaining stable blood sugar levels.

• Strategies for Decoding Carbs in Diabetes

1. Reading Food Labels:

   - Learn to decipher food labels, paying attention to the total carbohydrate content, and identifying sources of added sugars. This skill empowers you to make informed choices while grocery shopping.

2. Understanding Portion Sizes:

   - Portion control is a fundamental aspect of carb management. Recognizing appropriate portion sizes helps regulate carbohydrate intake, contributing to more stable blood sugar levels.

3. Choosing Whole Foods:

- Opt for whole, unprocessed foods that are rich in nutrients and fiber. Whole grains, fruits, and vegetables provide a more sustained release of glucose, supporting better blood sugar control.

4. Balancing Carbs with Proteins and Fats:

- Incorporate a balance of carbohydrates, proteins, and healthy fats in your meals. This combination helps slow down the absorption of glucose, preventing sudden spikes in blood sugar levels.

• Crafting a Diabetes-Friendly Diet

Decoding carbs in the context of diabetes involves crafting a diet that aligns with individual health goals. It's not about complete elimination but rather making smart choices and embracing a balanced approach.

• Personalizing Your Approach

Understanding that each person's experience with diabetes is unique, it's crucial to personalize your approach to carb management. Factors such as age, activity level, and overall health contribute to individualized dietary needs. Collaborating with healthcare professionals helps tailor a diabetes management plan that suits your specific requirements.

• Navigating the Grocery Aisles: Smart Shopping Strategies

The journey to decoding carbs starts at the grocery store. Armed with knowledge, navigating the aisles becomes a strategic endeavor. Adopting smart shopping strategies ensures that your cart is filled with foods conducive to diabetes management.

1. Focus on Fresh Produce:
   - Prioritize fresh fruits and vegetables. These nutrient-rich, low-calorie options are essential for a well-rounded and diabetes-friendly diet.

2. Whole Grains Matter:

- Choose whole grains over refined grains. Whole grains like brown rice, quinoa, and whole wheat provide more fiber, contributing to better blood sugar control.

3. Mindful Reading of Food Labels:

- Develop the habit of scrutinizing food labels. Look out for added sugars, and be wary of products that may seem healthy but hide hidden sugars.

• The Art of Meal Planning: Designing Diabetes-Friendly Menus

Meal planning emerges as a practical strategy in the journey to decode carbs for diabetes management. It involves thoughtful consideration of the types and amounts of foods consumed at each meal, ensuring a balanced and nutrient-dense approach.

1. Balancing Macronutrients:

- Construct meals that balance carbohydrates with proteins and healthy fats. This not only aids in blood sugar control but also provides sustained energy.

2. Explore Recipe Modifications:

- Transform favorite recipes into diabetes-friendly versions. Simple modifications, such as using whole-grain flour or reducing added sugars, can make a significant difference.

3. Batch Cooking for Convenience:

- Simplify meal preparation with batch cooking. This time-saving strategy ensures that you have nutritious and diabetes-friendly meals readily available.

• Beyond Restriction: Exploring Carb Alternatives

Decoding carbs isn't synonymous with restriction; it's about exploring alternatives that align with diabetes management goals. Discovering tasty substitutes for traditional high-carb ingredients adds variety to the diet while supporting blood sugar control.

1. Smart Swaps:
   - Experiment with smart swaps in your favorite recipes. For instance,

cauliflower rice can replace traditional rice, offering a lower-carb alternative.

2. Herbs and Spices for Flavor:
   - Embrace the world of herbs and spices to add flavor to your meals. Not only do they enhance taste, but some spices may also have potential health benefits.

• Embracing Wellness Beyond Carbs

Decoding carbs is just one facet of diabetes management. True wellness extends beyond dietary choices to encompass holistic health practices. Embracing mindful eating, incorporating regular exercise, managing stress, and prioritizing quality sleep contribute to an overall sense of wellbeing.

1. Mindful Eating Practices:
   - Cultivate mindful eating habits by paying attention to hunger and fullness cues. This practice fosters a healthier relationship with food and aids in better blood sugar control.

2. Physical Activity as a Pillar:
   - Integrate regular exercise into your routine. Physical activity not only supports blood sugar management but also contributes to overall cardiovascular health.

3. Stress Management Techniques:
   - Explore stress management techniques such as meditation or deep

breathing exercises. Chronic stress can impact blood sugar levels, and adopting stress-reducing practices is beneficial.

4. Prioritizing Quality Sleep:
   - Recognize the importance of quality sleep in diabetes management. Lack of sleep can affect insulin sensitivity, making adequate rest a crucial aspect of overall wellness.

• Your Journey to Decoding Carbs: A Path of Cultivating Healthy Habits

As you navigate the intricacies of decoding carbs in the context of diabetes, cultivating healthy habits becomes a focal point. Understanding your body's signals, acknowledging the impact of different foods and activities on blood sugar levels, and implementing small, sustainable changes contribute to a path of long-term success.

1. Understanding Body Signals:

- Listen to your body's signals. Recognize how different foods affect your blood sugar levels, and learn to make adjustments accordingly.

2. Implementing Small Changes Gradually:

- Sustainable changes often begin with small, manageable adjustments. Implementing these changes gradually allows for better adaptation and long-term success.

• Celebrating Progress: Recognizing the Power of Milestones

In the journey to decode carbs and manage diabetes effectively, celebrating progress, no matter how small, is a powerful motivator. Each milestone achieved is a testament to the positive impact of informed choices and healthy habits.

1. Acknowledging Achievements:
   - Take the time to acknowledge and celebrate achievements along the way. Whether it's reaching a weight loss goal or consistently maintaining stable blood sugar levels, every success is significant.

2. Motivating Continued Effort:

- Recognizing progress not only reinforces positive habits but also motivates continued effort. It instills confidence in your ability to manage diabetes effectively.

• Decoding Carbs for Diabetes Wellness

As we conclude this in-depth exploration of decoding carbs in the context of diabetes, the overarching theme is one of empowerment. Understanding the impact of carbohydrates on blood sugar levels, making informed choices, and embracing a balanced, personalized approach lays the foundation for effective diabetes management.

Decoding carbs is not a rigid process of restriction but a journey of exploration and adaptation. It's about making choices that align with your health goals, recognizing the significance of overall wellness, and cultivating habits that contribute to a vibrant and fulfilling life. In the intricate dance between carbs and diabetes, the power to decode lies in your hands, shaping a future marked by informed choices, balance, and optimal health.

CHAPTER 1

WHY CARBS MATTER

*T*he Foundations of Nutrition

To understand why carbs matter, let's begin with the basics of nutrition. Our bodies need various nutrients to function properly, and one of these key components is carbohydrates. Carbs serve as a primary source of energy, fueling our daily activities and bodily functions. They are one of the three main macronutrients, alongside proteins and fats.

• The Energy Currency of the Body

Imagine your body as a high-performance vehicle, and carbs as the fuel that keeps it running. When you consume carbohydrates, your digestive system breaks them down into glucose, a type of sugar. This glucose then enters your bloodstream, providing a readily available source of energy for your cells.

• Simple vs. Complex Carbs

Not all carbs are created equal. They come in two main types: simple and complex. Simple carbs, found in sugary snacks and beverages, provide a quick burst of energy. However, this energy is short-lived, often followed by a rapid drop in blood sugar levels.

On the other hand, complex carbs, present in whole grains, fruits, and vegetables, release energy more gradually. They offer a sustained fuel source, preventing the sudden energy spikes and crashes associated with simple carbs.

• Carbs and Blood Sugar Regulation

Now that we understand the role of carbs as an energy source, let's explore their connection to blood sugar regulation. Maintaining stable blood sugar levels is crucial for overall health, especially for individuals with conditions like diabetes.

• The Blood Sugar Roller Coaster

When you consume carbs, especially those high in simple sugars, your blood sugar levels can spike. This rapid increase triggers the release of insulin, a hormone that helps cells absorb glucose for energy. While this process is natural, frequent and extreme fluctuations in blood sugar levels can have adverse effects.

• Glycemic Index (GI) as a Guide

Enter the glycemic index (GI) – a tool that measures how quickly a carbohydrate-containing food raises blood sugar levels. Foods with a high GI cause a rapid spike, while those with a low GI release glucose more gradually. Understanding the GI helps in making informed choices, especially for individuals looking to manage their blood sugar levels effectively.

• The Brain's Preferred Fuel

Carbs aren't just energy for the body; they are also the preferred fuel for the brain. Unlike other organs, the brain relies almost exclusively on glucose for energy. When you consume carbs, they are broken down into glucose, providing a steady supply to keep your brain functioning optimally.

• Cognitive Function and Mood

Have you ever noticed feeling foggy or irritable when hungry? This could be attributed to low blood sugar levels. Consuming the right types of carbs can help maintain a steady supply of glucose to the brain, supporting cognitive function and mood stability.

• The Importance of Fiber

Many complex carbs, such as those found in whole grains and vegetables, are rich in fiber. Fiber not only contributes to digestive health but also slows down the absorption of glucose.

This gradual release helps avoid sudden spikes in blood sugar levels, promoting overall stability.

• Carbs as Building Blocks

Carbs go beyond being just a source of energy; they also play a role in building and maintaining various structures within the body.

• Cellular Structure and Function

Carbohydrates are integral components of cell membranes. They contribute to the structure and stability of cell walls, influencing how cells interact with their environment. This structural role is fundamental for the proper functioning of cells throughout the body.

• Glycoproteins and Glycolipids

Ever heard of glycoproteins and glycolipids? These are molecules consisting of carbohydrates and proteins or lipids. They play essential roles in cell communication, immune function, and various physiological processes. Carbs, in this context, act as building blocks for these crucial molecules.

• Carbs and Physical Performance

Whether you're an athlete or just trying to stay active, the role of carbohydrates in physical performance is undeniable. Carbs are the primary fuel source for muscles during exercise.

• Stored Energy in Muscles

When you eat carbs, your body converts them into glycogen, a form of stored energy in muscles and the liver. During physical activity, especially high-intensity exercise, your muscles rely on glycogen to sustain energy levels.

• Endurance and Recovery

For endurance activities like running or cycling, maintaining glycogen stores becomes critical. Consuming carbs before, during, and after exercise helps support endurance and enhances recovery by replenishing glycogen stores.

• Balancing Carbs with a Healthy Diet

Understanding why carbs matter leads us to the importance of balance in our overall diet. While carbs are essential, it's crucial to maintain a balanced intake of all nutrients.

• Balancing Macronutrients

A well-rounded diet includes a balance of carbohydrates, proteins, and fats. Each macronutrient plays a unique role in supporting bodily functions, and an imbalance can lead to various health issues.

• Micro and Macronutrient Harmony

In addition to macronutrients, a healthy diet includes essential micronutrients like vitamins and minerals. Balancing both macronutrients and micronutrients ensures that your body receives the necessary building blocks for optimal functioning.

• Carbs in Various Dietary Approaches

Carbs fit into various dietary approaches, each catering to different health goals and preferences.

• Low-Carb Diets

Some individuals opt for low-carb diets for weight management or blood sugar control. While reducing certain carbs, especially refined sugars, can be beneficial, it's essential to maintain a balance and choose nutrient-dense options.

• Carb Cycling

For those engaging in high-intensity workouts, carb cycling is a strategy where carb intake varies on different days. This approach aims to optimize glycogen stores for exercise performance.

• Plant-Based Diets

Plant-based diets, rich in fruits, vegetables, and whole grains, emphasize complex carbs. This dietary approach not only provides energy but also offers a wealth of vitamins, minerals, and antioxidants.

• Practical Tips for Smart Carb Choices

Now that we've explored the significance of carbs, let's conclude with practical tips for making smart carb choices in your daily life.

• Prioritize Whole Foods

Choose whole, unprocessed foods over refined and processed options. Whole grains, fruits, vegetables, and legumes provide a more extensive range of nutrients and fiber.

• Mindful Eating Habits

Practice mindful eating by paying attention to hunger and fullness cues. Eating slowly and savoring your food can help prevent overeating and promote a healthier relationship with food.

• Experiment with Carb Alternatives

Explore alternatives to refined carbs. For example, substitute sweet potatoes for regular potatoes or try cauliflower rice instead of traditional rice. These alternatives offer variety while contributing to a balanced diet.

• Stay Hydrated

Hydration is key to overall health. Drink water regularly, especially if you consume a higher-fiber diet, as fiber absorbs water. Proper hydration supports digestion and helps maintain optimal bodily functions.

• Consult with Healthcare Professionals

If you have specific health goals or medical conditions, consult with healthcare professionals, including a registered dietitian or nutritionist. They can provide personalized guidance based on your unique needs.

• The Carbohydrate Tapestry

In unraveling the question of why carbs matter, we discover that carbohydrates are not just sources of energy; they are intricately woven into the fabric of our health. From fueling our brain and muscles to serving as building blocks for essential molecules, carbs play diverse roles that impact every aspect of our well-being.

The key lies in understanding the nuances of carbs, making informed choices, and embracing a balanced approach to nutrition. Carbs matter because they are fundamental to our vitality, supporting us in our daily activities, cognitive function, and overall health journey. As you navigate the carbohydrate tapestry of your diet, may your choices be guided by knowledge, balance, and a commitment to nourishing your body for a vibrant and healthy life.

✓ Going Deeper into the Basics

• The ABCs of Nutrition

Let's dive deep into the basics of nutrition, starting with the ABCs. Nutrition is like the instruction manual for our body, and understanding it helps us make choices that keep everything running smoothly.

• Macronutrients: The Big Three

Macronutrients are the nutrients our bodies need in large amounts. There are three main players: carbohydrates, proteins, and fats. Carbs provide energy, proteins build and repair tissues, and fats support cell function. Imagine them as the fuel, builders, and maintainers of your body.

• Micronutrients: Tiny Heroes

Micronutrients are like the unsung heroes, needed in smaller amounts but equally crucial. These include vitamins and minerals that play various roles, from keeping our skin healthy to helping us see in the dark.

• Carbs - More Than Just Energy

Carbohydrates, or carbs, are often seen as the energy superheroes. But there's more to them than just fuel.

Carbs come in two forms: simple and complex. Simple carbs are like sprinters, providing a quick burst of energy found in sugary treats. Complex carbs, found in whole grains and veggies, are more like marathon runners, releasing energy steadily over time.

• Fiber: The Digestive Hero

Enter fiber, an essential part of many complex carbs. Fiber is like the traffic manager for your digestive system, keeping things moving smoothly. It's found in fruits, veggies, and whole grains and helps prevent constipation.

• Protein - Builders of the Body

Proteins are the builders, responsible for constructing and repairing tissues.

• Amino Acids: The Building Blocks

Proteins are made up of amino acids, like Lego pieces building different structures. There are essential amino acids our bodies can't make, so we need to get them from our diet.

• Protein's Many Roles

Proteins aren't just for muscles; they play a part in creating enzymes for digestion, antibodies for our immune system, and even acting as messengers in our cells.

• Fats - The Supportive Sidekick

Fats are often misunderstood, but they're crucial for various bodily functions.

- Types of Fats: Friends and Foes

Not all fats are the same. There are healthy fats, like those found in avocados and nuts, and unhealthy fats, like those in fried foods. Healthy fats are like the support crew, aiding in nutrient absorption and protecting our organs.

• Omega-3 Fatty Acids: Brain Boosters

Ever heard of omega-3s? They're a type of healthy fat that's like a superhero for your brain, supporting cognitive function and mood.

• Vitamins and Minerals - The Micronutrient Team

Vitamins and minerals may be needed in smaller amounts, but they are mighty in their impact.

• Vitamins: Boosters and Protectors

Vitamins act like boosters for various bodily functions. Vitamin C, for example, boosts our immune system, while vitamin D helps our bodies absorb calcium for strong bones.

• Minerals: The Silent Supporters

Minerals, like calcium and iron, play crucial roles. Calcium is like the construction worker, building strong bones and teeth, while iron is the courier, delivering oxygen throughout the body.

• Water - The Unsung Hero

Water often doesn't get the credit it deserves, but it's the unsung hero in our nutritional story.

• Hydration: More Than Just a Drink

Water is essential for almost every bodily function. It's like the liquid transporter, moving nutrients, and aiding in digestion. Staying hydrated helps keep our skin healthy and supports our joints.

• Dehydration: The Villain

Not getting enough water can lead to dehydration, the villain in our story. It can cause fatigue, dizziness, and even impact our mood. So, keep that water bottle handy!

• Putting It All Together - The Balanced Plate

Now that we know about the ABCs and superheroes of nutrition, how do we create a balanced plate?

• The Balanced Plate: A Visual Guide

Imagine your plate as a canvas, and you're the artist. Fill half of it with colorful veggies and fruits, one-quarter with whole grains or starchy veggies, and the remaining quarter with protein-rich foods. This creates a balanced and nutritious masterpiece.

• Moderation: The Key Ingredient

The key to a balanced plate is moderation. It's like the conductor in an orchestra, ensuring that no nutrient takes over the spotlight.

• Listening to Your Body - The Ultimate Guide

The final chapter is about tuning in to what your body needs. It's like having a personalized guide to your own well-being.

• Hunger and Fullness: Your Body's Signals

Pay attention to your body's signals of hunger and fullness. It's like having a built-in GPS, guiding you to when and how much to eat.

Cravings: Messages from Within

Cravings aren't always the enemy. They can be messages from your body, indicating a need for specific nutrients. So, instead of fighting them, decode the messages they bring.

Adaptability: Your Body, Your Guide

Our bodies are incredibly adaptable. Listen to how it responds to different foods and adjust your choices accordingly. It's like having a personal coach, giving you feedback on what works best.

Intuitive Eating: Trusting Your Instincts

Embrace intuitive eating, a practice of trusting your body to guide your food choices. It's like having a wise friend, helping you navigate the vast world of nutrition with confidence.

• Your Nutritional Journey

You've gone deeper into the basics of nutrition, discovering the superheroes of the food world. Remember, nutrition isn't about perfection but progress. So, whether you're savoring the role of carbs, appreciating the builders (proteins), or understanding the supportive sidekick (fats), know that your nutritional journey is uniquely yours. Embrace it, savor it, and nourish your body for a vibrant and healthy life.

CHAPTER 2

BUILDING YOUR PERSONAL DIABETES PLAN

Embarking on the journey of building a personal diabetes plan is a transformative process that empowers individuals to take control of their health and well-being. Crafting a plan tailored to your unique needs involves a comprehensive understanding of diabetes, lifestyle choices, and a commitment to sustainable, positive change. As we delve into the intricacies of building your personal diabetes plan, envision this as a roadmap – a guide that aligns with your goals, preferences, and the realities of your everyday life.

• Understanding Diabetes:

The foundation of your personal diabetes plan lies in a clear understanding of diabetes itself. Diabetes is a condition characterized by elevated blood sugar levels due to the body's inability to produce enough insulin or effectively use the insulin it produces. Insulin, a hormone produced by the pancreas, regulates the absorption of glucose into cells for energy. Without proper insulin function, glucose accumulates in the bloodstream, leading to high blood sugar levels.

• Types of Diabetes:

There are primarily two types of diabetes: Type 1 and Type 2. Type 1 diabetes is an autoimmune condition where the immune system attacks and destroys insulin-producing cells in the pancreas. Individuals with Type 1 diabetes rely on insulin injections for life.

Type 2 diabetes, on the other hand, is more common and often associated with lifestyle factors. It occurs when the body becomes resistant to the effects of insulin or doesn't produce enough insulin to maintain normal blood sugar levels. Lifestyle modifications, including diet and physical activity, play a crucial role in managing Type 2 diabetes.

• Building Awareness:

The first step in crafting your personal diabetes plan is to build awareness. Understand your specific type of diabetes, its potential complications, and how it uniquely manifests in your body. Regular monitoring of blood sugar levels provides valuable insights into how your body responds to different foods, activities, and medications.

• Collaboration with Healthcare Professionals:

Your healthcare team becomes an essential ally in constructing your diabetes plan. Engage with your primary care physician, endocrinologist, dietitian, and other specialists as needed. Regular check-ups and open communication establish a collaborative relationship, ensuring that your plan aligns with your health goals and adapts to any changes in your condition.

• Lifestyle Factors in Diabetes Management:

Nutrition:

Central to your diabetes plan is a thoughtful approach to nutrition. Rather than viewing it as a restrictive diet, think of it as a way to nourish your body and manage blood sugar levels effectively.

1. Carbohydrate Management:

- Understand the impact of carbohydrates on blood sugar levels. Learn to differentiate between simple and complex carbs and explore the concept of the glycemic index (GI), which measures how quickly a food raises blood sugar.

- Practice portion control to manage carb intake. Balancing your meals with a mix of carbs, proteins, and healthy fats contributes to stable blood sugar levels.

2. Whole Foods Emphasis:

- Prioritize whole, unprocessed foods rich in fiber, vitamins, and minerals. Vegetables, fruits, whole grains, and lean proteins form the foundation of a nutrient-dense diet.

3. Regular Meal Timing:

- Establish consistent meal timings to regulate blood sugar levels. Avoid skipping meals, and consider spreading your daily food intake across smaller, balanced meals and snacks.

• Physical Activity:

Incorporating regular physical activity into your routine is a powerful component of diabetes management.

1. Aerobic Exercise:

- Engage in aerobic exercises like walking, jogging, cycling, or swimming. These activities help improve insulin sensitivity and contribute to overall cardiovascular health.

2. Strength Training:

- Include strength training exercises to build and maintain muscle mass. Muscle tissue plays a role in glucose metabolism, assisting in blood sugar control.

3. Flexibility and Balance:

- Incorporate flexibility and balance exercises, such as yoga or tai chi, to enhance overall well-being. These activities contribute to joint health and may positively impact blood sugar levels.

• Stress Management:

Chronic stress can affect blood sugar levels, and therefore, effective stress management is an integral part of your diabetes plan.

1. Mindfulness Practices:
   - Explore mindfulness techniques like meditation, deep breathing exercises, or guided imagery. These practices can help reduce stress levels and promote a sense of calm.

2. Time for Relaxation:
   - Allocate time for activities that bring you joy and relaxation. Whether it's

reading, spending time in nature, or pursuing hobbies, these moments contribute to overall stress reduction.

• Adequate Sleep:

Quality sleep is essential for overall health, and its impact on blood sugar levels should not be underestimated.

1. Establish a Sleep Routine:
   - Create a consistent sleep schedule, aiming for 7-9 hours of quality sleep each night. Going to bed and waking up at the same time each day helps regulate your body's internal clock.

2. Sleep Environment:
   - Create a comfortable sleep environment by keeping your bedroom

dark, quiet, and cool. Limit screen time before bedtime to promote better sleep quality.

• Hydration:

Proper hydration is often overlooked but plays a crucial role in supporting overall health and diabetes management.

1. Regular Water Intake:
   - Drink an adequate amount of water throughout the day. Staying hydrated supports kidney function, aids digestion, and may help regulate blood sugar levels.

2. Limit Sugary Beverages:

- Avoid sugary beverages, as they can lead to rapid spikes in blood sugar. Opt for water, herbal teas, or infused water for refreshing, low-calorie alternatives.

• Medication Adherence:

If prescribed medication as part of your diabetes management plan, consistent adherence is vital.

1. Understand Your Medications:
    - Familiarize yourself with your medications, including their purpose, dosage, and potential side effects. If you have any concerns or questions, discuss them with your healthcare provider.

2. Adhere to Prescribed Schedule:

- Take medications as prescribed, adhering to the recommended schedule. Set reminders or use pill organizers to help ensure consistency.

• Regular Monitoring and Adjustment:

Effective diabetes management involves ongoing monitoring and the flexibility to adjust your plan as needed.

1. Blood Sugar Monitoring:
   - Regularly monitor your blood sugar levels as recommended by your healthcare provider. Keeping a log or using digital tools helps track patterns and facilitates informed discussions with your healthcare team.

2. Health Check-ups:

- Attend regular check-ups with your healthcare team. These appointments provide opportunities to discuss any challenges, make adjustments to your plan, and address emerging health concerns.

• Emotional Well-being:

Recognizing the emotional aspects of living with diabetes is essential for holistic well-being.

1. Support System:
   - Build a support system that may include family, friends, or diabetes support groups. Sharing experiences and challenges fosters a sense of community and emotional well-being.

2. Mental Health Awareness:
   - Be mindful of your mental health. If you experience symptoms of anxiety or depression, seek support from mental health professionals. Emotional well-being is interconnected with overall health.

• Cultural Considerations:

Acknowledge and incorporate cultural factors into your diabetes plan.

1. Traditional Foods:
   - Explore ways to include traditional foods in your diet, making adjustments for their impact on blood sugar levels. This approach adds cultural richness to your meals.

2. Community Engagement:

- Engage with community resources that align with your cultural background. Community events, workshops, or support groups can provide valuable insights and a sense of belonging.

• Financial Considerations:

Consider the financial aspects of your diabetes plan.

1. Affordable Food Choices:

- Make informed, affordable choices when it comes to food. Emphasize cost-effective, nutrient-dense options that support your overall health.

2. Medication Accessibility:

- Ensure access to prescribed medications. If financial constraints are a concern, communicate openly with your healthcare team to explore affordable alternatives or assistance programs.

• Lifelong Learning:

View diabetes management as a journey of lifelong learning.

1. Stay Informed:

- Stay informed about the latest advancements in diabetes management. Attend educational events, read reputable sources, and remain curious about new strategies or technologies that may benefit you.

2. Adapt and Evolve:

- Embrace a mindset of adaptation and evolution. As your life circumstances, health, and medical knowledge evolve, be open to adjusting your diabetes plan to reflect these changes.

• Celebrating Successes:
Acknowledge and celebrate your successes along the way.

1. Milestones and Achievements:

- Celebrate both small and significant milestones. Whether it's achieving a target blood sugar level, maintaining a consistent exercise routine, or making positive dietary changes, each success contributes to your overall well-being.

2. Positive Reinforcement:

- Provide yourself with positive reinforcement. Recognize the effort you invest in your diabetes plan and the positive impact it has on your health. Cultivate a mindset of self-appreciation.

In essence, building your personal diabetes plan is a holistic endeavor that integrates various aspects of your life. It is a dynamic, adaptable process that recognizes your individuality and emphasizes the interconnectedness of physical, emotional, and lifestyle factors.

✓ Setting the Foundations

Setting the foundations for a healthy and fulfilling life involves establishing habits, routines, and mindset shifts that contribute to overall well-being. Think of this process as laying the groundwork for a sturdy structure, one that supports you physically, mentally, and emotionally.

• Understanding Your Starting Point:

The first step in setting foundations is gaining clarity on your current lifestyle, habits, and overall health. This self-awareness serves as the cornerstone upon which you can build positive changes. Reflect on your daily routines, dietary choices, physical activity, stress levels, and sleep patterns. Take note of areas where you excel and identify areas for improvement.

• Health Assessment:

Consider undergoing a comprehensive health assessment to understand your baseline health. This may include blood tests, body measurements, and discussions with healthcare professionals. Understanding key health indicators provides valuable insights into areas that may require attention and guides the development of personalized goals.

• Defining Your Values and Priorities:

Clarify your values and priorities to guide your journey. What matters most to you? Is it physical health, mental well-being, relationships, or personal growth? By aligning your goals with your values, you create a sense of purpose that fuels your commitment to positive change.

• Mindset Shifts:

Cultivate a growth mindset that embraces challenges and views setbacks as opportunities for learning and improvement. Adopting a positive and resilient mindset is foundational to overcoming obstacles and staying motivated on your wellness journey.

• Building a Support System:

Recognize the importance of a strong support system. Share your goals with friends, family, or like-minded individuals who can provide encouragement, accountability, and understanding. Building a community around your health aspirations enhances your ability to stay on track and navigate challenges.

• Nutrition as a Foundation:

The food you consume is a fundamental building block for your health. Approach nutrition as nourishment, focusing on whole, nutrient-dense foods that support your body's functions.

1. Balanced Diet:
   - Strive for a balanced diet that includes a variety of fruits, vegetables, whole grains, lean proteins, and healthy fats. This diversity ensures that your body receives essential nutrients for optimal functioning.

2. Portion Control:

- Practice portion control to avoid overeating. Pay attention to hunger and fullness cues, and savor your meals mindfully. Portion control contributes to maintaining a healthy weight and preventing overconsumption of calories.

3. Hydration:

- Prioritize hydration by drinking an adequate amount of water throughout the day. Water supports digestion, nutrient absorption, and overall bodily functions. Limit sugary beverages and opt for water as your primary hydration source.

4. Mindful Eating:

- Embrace mindful eating practices. Slow down during meals, savor each bite, and pay attention to the flavors and textures of your food. Mindful eating fosters a healthier relationship with food and prevents mindless overeating.

• Physical Activity as a Pillar:

Incorporate regular physical activity into your routine to strengthen your body, enhance mood, and support overall health.

1. Find Activities You Enjoy:
   - Engage in physical activities that bring you joy. Whether it's dancing, hiking, cycling, or yoga, choosing activities you enjoy increases the likelihood of consistent participation.

2. Consistency Over Intensity:

- Prioritize consistency over intensity. Establish a realistic and sustainable exercise routine that aligns with your preferences and fits into your schedule. Regular, moderate exercise often yields more sustainable benefits than sporadic intense workouts.

3. Mix Cardiovascular and Strength Training:

- Include a mix of cardiovascular exercises and strength training. Cardiovascular activities enhance heart health and burn calories, while strength training supports muscle development and metabolism.

• Stress Management Techniques:

Acknowledge the impact of stress on your well-being and implement effective stress management techniques.

1. Mindfulness and Meditation:
    - Incorporate mindfulness and meditation into your daily routine. These practices help reduce stress, improve focus, and cultivate a sense of calm. Begin with short sessions and gradually increase the duration as you build the habit.

2. Deep Breathing Exercises:
    - Practice deep breathing exercises to activate the body's relaxation response. Deep, intentional breaths can be a quick and effective tool to manage stress in various situations.

3. Establish Boundaries:

   - Set clear boundaries to manage stressors in your life. Learning to say no when necessary and prioritizing self-care contribute to a healthier balance between responsibilities and personal well-being.

• Quality Sleep:

Recognize the importance of quality sleep in supporting physical and mental health.

1. Consistent Sleep Schedule:

   - Establish a consistent sleep schedule by going to bed and waking up at the same time each day. Consistency regulates your body's internal clock and promotes better sleep quality.

2. Create a Relaxing Bedtime Routine:
   - Develop a relaxing bedtime routine to signal to your body that it's time to wind down. Avoid stimulating activities and screens close to bedtime, opting for calming rituals such as reading or gentle stretching.

3. Optimize Sleep Environment:
   - Create an optimal sleep environment. Keep your bedroom dark, quiet, and cool. Invest in a comfortable mattress and pillows to support restful sleep.

• Mindfulness and Emotional Well-being:

Nurture your emotional well-being through mindfulness practices and self-awareness.

1. Journaling:

- Incorporate journaling into your routine. Reflect on your thoughts, emotions, and experiences. Journaling provides an outlet for self-expression and can enhance self-awareness.

2. Gratitude Practices:

- Cultivate gratitude by acknowledging and appreciating positive aspects of your life. Practicing gratitude can shift your focus towards positive experiences and contribute to a more optimistic mindset.

• Continual Learning and Growth:

View life as a journey of continual learning and growth. Embrace new opportunities, seek knowledge, and be open to personal development.

1. Set Learning Goals:
   - Establish learning goals alongside your health and well-being goals. Whether it's acquiring a new skill, exploring a hobby, or pursuing educational opportunities, a commitment to learning fosters a sense of purpose.

2. Adaptability:
   - Cultivate adaptability as a core skill. Life is dynamic, and being adaptable allows you to navigate challenges with

resilience. Embrace change as an opportunity for growth rather than a source of stress.

• Financial Well-being:

Consider the financial aspects of your life and make intentional choices that align with your values.

1. Budgeting:
   - Create a budget that reflects your financial goals and priorities. Tracking your expenses and saving for future needs contribute to financial stability.

2. Emergency Fund:
   - Build an emergency fund to provide a financial safety net. Having savings set aside for unexpected expenses

reduces stress and enhances your overall financial well-being.

• Social Connections:

Acknowledge the importance of social connections in fostering a sense of belonging and support.

1. Quality Relationships:
   - Cultivate quality relationships with friends and family. Invest time in meaningful connections that contribute positively to your life.

2. Community Engagement:
   - Engage with your community through social activities, volunteering, or joining clubs or groups. Building a sense of community strengthens your

support network and enhances overall well-being.

• Cultural Considerations:

Integrate your cultural background into your daily life and well-being practices.

1. Traditional Practices:
   - Incorporate traditional practices and cultural celebrations into your routine. This connection to your cultural heritage adds richness to your life.

2. Community Involvement:
   - Participate in community events that celebrate your cultural identity. Engaging with your cultural community provides a sense of belonging and

fosters a deeper connection to your roots.

• Celebrating Progress:

Acknowledge and celebrate your progress, no matter how small. Regularly revisit your goals, assess your achievements, and express gratitude for the positive changes you've implemented.

1. Reflection:
   - Take time for reflection on a regular basis. Reflecting on your journey allows you to appreciate your growth, identify areas for further improvement, and adjust your approach as needed.

2. Reward Yourself:

- Establish a system of rewards for reaching milestones. Whether it's treating yourself to a favorite activity or acknowledging your achievements with a small celebration, positive reinforcement enhances motivation.

• Adapting to Change:

Recognize that change is a constant in life, and your foundations should be adaptable to evolving circumstances.

1. Flexibility:
- Embrace flexibility in your routines and plans. Being adaptable allows you to navigate unexpected changes without feeling overwhelmed.

2. Learn from Setbacks:

- View setbacks as opportunities for learning and growth. Instead of dwelling on challenges, extract lessons that can inform your future decisions and actions.

In summary, setting the foundations for a healthy and fulfilling life involves a holistic approach that addresses physical, mental, emotional, and lifestyle aspects. This blueprint is not rigid but adaptable, reflecting the dynamic nature of life.

✓ Making It Work for You

Making your health and well-being strategies work for you is a dynamic process that involves tailoring lifestyle changes to your individual preferences, circumstances, and goals. It's about creating a sustainable and personalized approach that aligns with your unique needs.

• Understanding Individuality:

Recognizing and embracing your individuality is the first step in making health strategies work for you. Everyone is unique, with different preferences, schedules, and challenges. What works for one person may not work for another. By acknowledging your individual traits, you lay the foundation for a customized approach that resonates with your life.

• Personalized Goal Setting:

Begin by setting personalized and realistic goals that align with your overarching vision for well-being. Consider both short-term and long-term objectives, ensuring they are specific, measurable, achievable, relevant, and time-bound (SMART). This strategic goal-setting approach provides clarity and direction.

• Tailoring Nutrition to Your Tastes:

Nutrition is a cornerstone of well-being, and tailoring your dietary choices to your tastes is key to long-term success.

1. Explore Healthy Food Options:
   - Experiment with a variety of nutritious foods to discover what you enjoy. The world of healthy eating is

vast, encompassing a rich array of fruits, vegetables, whole grains, lean proteins, and healthy fats. Find combinations that appeal to your taste buds.

2. Adapt Traditional Recipes:

- If you have cultural or familial dietary preferences, adapt traditional recipes to make them more health-conscious. Substitute ingredients, focus on whole foods, and experiment with herbs and spices to enhance flavor without relying on excessive salt or sugar.

3. Mindful Eating Practices:

- Incorporate mindful eating practices into your routine. Pay attention to hunger and fullness cues, savor each bite, and eat without distractions. This approach not only enhances your connection to the food but also promotes a healthier relationship with eating.

• Fitness That Fits Your Lifestyle:

Finding a fitness routine that fits seamlessly into your lifestyle is crucial for consistency and enjoyment.

1. Identify Activities You Enjoy:
   - Explore physical activities that align with your interests. Whether it's dancing, hiking, swimming, or team sports, choose exercises that bring you joy. When you enjoy the activity, it becomes a sustainable part of your routine.

2. Incorporate Into Daily Life:

   - Integrate exercise into your daily life. This could involve walking or biking to work, taking the stairs instead of the elevator, or incorporating short bursts of physical activity throughout the day. These small adjustments accumulate and contribute to overall fitness.

3. Flexibility in Routine:

   - Embrace flexibility in your fitness routine. Life is dynamic, and there will be times when your usual workout may not be feasible. Having alternative activities or shorter workout options allows you to adapt without feeling discouraged.

• Stress Management Strategies:

Developing effective stress management strategies is essential for maintaining overall well-being.

1. Identify Stress Triggers:
    - Identify your stress triggers. Understanding the sources of stress empowers you to implement targeted strategies. Whether it's work-related pressures, personal relationships, or external factors, recognizing triggers is the first step in managing stress.

2. Incorporate Relaxation Techniques:
    - Integrate relaxation techniques into your daily routine. This may include mindfulness meditation, deep breathing exercises, or progressive muscle

relaxation. These practices can be tailored to suit your preferences and time constraints.

3. Establish Boundaries:

- Set clear boundaries to manage stressors effectively. Learn to say no when necessary, prioritize self-care, and create a balance between responsibilities and personal well-being. Establishing boundaries is an ongoing process that evolves as you navigate different life stages.

• Prioritizing Quality Sleep:

Quality sleep is a cornerstone of health, and tailoring your sleep routine to suit your needs is crucial.

1. Consistent Sleep Schedule:

   - Establish a consistent sleep schedule that aligns with your natural circadian rhythm. Going to bed and waking up at the same time each day helps regulate your body's internal clock, promoting better sleep quality.

2. Create a Relaxing Bedtime Ritual:

   - Develop a relaxing bedtime ritual to signal to your body that it's time to wind down. This could involve activities such as reading, taking a warm bath, or practicing gentle stretches. Creating a calming pre-sleep routine prepares your mind and body for rest.

3. Optimize Sleep Environment:

   - Personalize your sleep environment for optimal comfort. This may include investing in a comfortable mattress and pillows, adjusting room temperature, and minimizing noise and light. Tailoring your sleep environment enhances the quality of your sleep.

• Mindfulness for Emotional Well-being:

Cultivating mindfulness practices contributes to emotional well-being and can be adapted to suit your lifestyle.

1. Find Your Mindfulness Outlet:
   - Explore different mindfulness practices to find what resonates with you. This could include meditation, guided imagery, mindful walking, or even mindful eating. Tailoring these

practices to your preferences enhances their effectiveness.

2. Incorporate Mindfulness Into Daily Activities:
   - Integrate mindfulness into your daily activities. This involves bringing your full attention to the present moment, whether you're eating, walking, or engaging in routine tasks. Mindful living promotes a sense of calm and clarity.

3. Adapt Mindfulness to Your Schedule:
   - Adapt mindfulness practices to your schedule. If time is limited, incorporate short mindfulness exercises into your day. These can be as brief as a few minutes but contribute significantly to

reducing stress and promoting emotional balance.

• Financial Wellness Strategies:

Addressing financial well-being involves tailoring strategies that align with your financial goals and lifestyle.

1. Create a Realistic Budget:
    - Develop a realistic budget that considers your income, expenses, and financial goals. A personalized budget reflects your priorities and allows for intentional spending.

2. Emergency Fund Planning:
    - Plan for financial emergencies by building an emergency fund. Having savings set aside provides a financial

safety net, reducing stress during unexpected situations.

3. Prioritize Investments:
    - Tailor your investment strategy to align with your financial objectives. Whether it's saving for retirement, a home, or education, personalized investment choices contribute to long-term financial stability.

• Social Connections:

Nurturing social connections involves adapting your interactions to suit your personality and preferences.

1. Quality Over Quantity:
    - Prioritize quality over quantity in your social connections. Cultivate

meaningful relationships with individuals who support and uplift you. Tailoring your social circle contributes to a positive and fulfilling social life.

2. Flexible Socializing:

- Be flexible in your socializing approach. If large gatherings are not your preference, consider one-on-one interactions or smaller group settings. Tailoring social activities to suit your comfort level enhances the enjoyment of social connections.

• Cultural Considerations:

Integrating cultural considerations into your well-being strategies involves celebrating your heritage in ways that resonate with you.

1. Traditional Practices:

- Incorporate traditional practices that hold personal significance. This could involve participating in cultural celebrations, preparing traditional foods, or engaging in rituals that connect you to your heritage.

2. Community Engagement:

- Engage with your cultural community in ways that align with your interests. Whether it's joining community events, participating in cultural organizations, or volunteering, integrating cultural aspects into your life adds richness and a sense of belonging.

• Celebrating Progress and Adjusting Strategies:

Regularly assess your progress and be open to adjusting your strategies based on evolving needs and circumstances.

1. Reflect on Achievements:
   - Take time to reflect on your achievements. Celebrate the progress you've made toward your goals, acknowledging both small and significant victories. Positive reinforcement enhances motivation.

2. Adaptation and Flexibility:
   - Embrace adaptability and flexibility in your strategies. Life is dynamic, and what worked at one point may need adjustment as circumstances change.

Being open to adaptation ensures that your well-being strategies remain relevant and effective.

In essence, making health and well-being strategies work for you is an ongoing and adaptive process. Tailoring your approach to your individual preferences, values, and life circumstances empowers you to create a sustainable lifestyle that promotes overall well-being.

CHAPTER 3

SMART GROCERY SHOPPING

Smart grocery shopping is a foundational skill that not only contributes to a well-balanced and nutritious diet but also helps you make informed choices that align with your health goals and budget.

• Understanding the Importance of Smart Grocery Shopping:

Before delving into the specifics of smart grocery shopping, it's essential to understand why this skill is crucial for your overall well-being. Smart grocery shopping is about more than just filling your cart with food; it's a strategic approach to nourishing your body, managing your budget, and making choices that support your health goals.

1. Nutrient-Rich Choices:

- Smart grocery shopping empowers you to choose nutrient-dense foods that provide essential vitamins, minerals, and other beneficial compounds. By prioritizing whole, unprocessed foods, you maximize the nutritional value of your meals.

2. Balanced Diet:

- It facilitates the creation of a balanced and varied diet. A diverse range of fruits, vegetables, whole grains, lean proteins, and healthy fats ensures that you receive a broad spectrum of nutrients, contributing to overall health.

3. Budget Management:

- Smart grocery shopping helps you manage your budget effectively. By planning, making strategic choices, and avoiding impulse purchases, you can optimize your spending while still meeting your nutritional needs.

4. Meal Planning:

- It supports meal planning and preparation. Knowing what ingredients to buy and having a plan for how to use them reduces food waste, saves time, and promotes healthier eating habits.

5. Label Awareness:

- Understanding food labels enables you to make informed decisions about the products you choose. This includes assessing nutritional content, ingredient lists, and marketing claims to ensure alignment with your health objectives.

• Before You Shop:

1. Create a Shopping List:
   - Begin your smart grocery shopping journey by creating a comprehensive shopping list. This not only helps you stay organized but also prevents unnecessary purchases and ensures you have all the ingredients you need for your meals.

2. Plan Your Meals:
   - Meal planning is a key component of smart grocery shopping. Take some time to plan your meals for the week, considering a balance of proteins,

carbohydrates, fats, and a variety of fruits and vegetables. This guides your list creation and helps you avoid last-minute, less-healthy choices.

3. Check Your Pantry:

- Before heading to the store, check your pantry, refrigerator, and freezer. Take note of items you already have to avoid purchasing duplicates. This reduces food waste and contributes to a more organized kitchen.

4. Set a Budget:

- Establish a realistic budget for your grocery shopping. Having a clear spending limit helps you make conscious choices and prevents overspending. Consider allocating a specific amount for different categories, such as produce, proteins, and pantry staples.

• Navigating the Aisles:

1. Start with Fresh Produce:
   - Begin your grocery shopping in the fresh produce section. Fill your cart with a colorful array of fruits and vegetables. These nutrient-packed foods form the foundation of a healthy diet and add variety to your meals.

   - Tips:
   - Choose a mix of colors to ensure a diverse range of nutrients.
        - Consider seasonal produce for freshness and cost-effectiveness.

- Be mindful of perishable items and plan meals accordingly to minimize waste.

2. Explore the Perimeter:
- The perimeter of the grocery store typically houses fresh produce, meats, dairy, and other whole foods. Spend a significant portion of your time in these areas, as they offer a wealth of nutritious options.

- Tips:
- Opt for lean proteins like chicken, turkey, fish, and plant-based options.
- Choose whole grains such as brown rice, quinoa, and whole wheat products.
- Explore different dairy or non-dairy alternatives based on your preferences.

3.   Navigate   the   Center   Aisles Mindfully:

- While many processed and less nutritious items are found in the center aisles, they also contain essential pantry staples. Approach these aisles with mindfulness, focusing on whole and minimally processed options.

- Tips:

- Read labels carefully and choose products with fewer additives.

- Prioritize whole grains, legumes, and canned goods without added sugars.

- Compare different brands for nutritional content and choose wisely.

4. Read and Decode Food Labels:

- Understanding food labels empowers you to make informed

choices. Pay attention to serving sizes, nutritional content, and ingredient lists. Look for products with recognizable, whole-food ingredients and minimal additives.

- Tips:

- Be wary of added sugars, excessive sodium, and artificial additives.

- Consider the order of ingredients – items are listed in descending order by weight.

- Familiarize yourself with key nutritional values like calories, protein, fiber, and vitamins.

5. Be Selective with Packaged Snacks:

- If you opt for packaged snacks, choose wisely. Look for options with minimal added sugars, healthy fats, and adequate protein. Whole-food snacks like nuts, seeds, and dried fruits can be nutritious choices.

- Tips:
- Check the ingredient list for hidden sugars and unhealthy fats.
- Choose snacks that provide sustained energy and satiety.
- Portion control is key – pre-portion snacks to avoid overeating.

6. Don't Shop Hungry:

- Shopping on an empty stomach can lead to impulsive, less healthy choices. Eat a balanced meal or snack before heading to the store to make rational decisions and avoid unnecessary purchases.

- Tips:

- Carry a water bottle to stay hydrated and curb hunger.

- Focus on your shopping list and stick to your planned purchases.

• Making Informed Choices:

1. Prioritize Whole, Unprocessed Foods:

- The foundation of smart grocery shopping is choosing whole, unprocessed foods. These include fresh produce, lean proteins, whole grains, and minimally processed dairy or dairy alternatives. These foods provide essential nutrients without added preservatives or artificial ingredients.

2. Choose Lean Proteins:

- Prioritize lean protein sources like poultry, fish, legumes, tofu, and low-fat dairy. These options provide essential amino acids for muscle health without excess saturated fats.

3. Opt for Whole Grains:

- Select whole grains like brown rice, quinoa, oats, and whole wheat products. Whole grains offer fiber, vitamins, and minerals, promoting digestive health and sustained energy.

4. Select Healthy Fats:

- Incorporate healthy fats into your cart, such as avocados, nuts, seeds, and olive oil. These fats contribute to heart health, provide satiety, and support the absorption of fat-soluble vitamins.

5. Mindful Beverage Choices:
  - Choose beverages mindfully. Opt for water as your primary hydrating source and limit sugary drinks. Herbal teas and infused water are refreshing alternatives without added calories.

6. Consider Frozen and Canned Options:
  - Frozen fruits and vegetables, as well as canned goods, can be convenient and nutritious options. Look for frozen vegetables without added sauces or canned goods with minimal preservatives.

7. Shop Seasonally:
  - Incorporate seasonal produce into your shopping list. Seasonal fruits and vegetables are often fresher, more

affordable, and offer variety throughout the year.

8. Be Mindful of Sales and Promotions:
   - While sales and promotions can save you money, be mindful of their impact on your choices. Avoid buying items solely because they are on sale if they don't align with your health goals or needs.

• Post-Shopping Tips:

1. Practice Safe Food Handling:
    - Once you're home, practice safe food handling to maintain the freshness and safety of your groceries. Store perishable items promptly, refrigerate or freeze as needed, and be mindful of expiration dates.

2. Prepare Meals in Advance:

- Use your smartly chosen groceries to prepare meals in advance. This reduces the likelihood of opting for less healthy, convenient options when time is limited.

3. Embrace Variety in Your Diet:

- Utilize the variety of foods you've purchased to create diverse and enjoyable meals. Embracing variety not only enhances your nutritional intake but also makes the eating experience more satisfying.

4. Reflect on Your Choices:

- Periodically reflect on your grocery shopping choices. Consider what worked well, what could be improved, and how your shopping habits align with your health goals. This reflective practice enhances your ability to make informed choices in the future.

5. Adjust Your Shopping List:

- Based on your reflections and evolving health goals, adjust your shopping list accordingly. Be open to trying new foods, recipes, and incorporating feedback from your own experiences.

Smart grocery shopping is a skill that evolves with practice and mindfulness. By approaching the process with a strategic mindset, understanding the nutritional value of foods, and aligning your choices with your health goals and budget, you can transform your grocery shopping experience into a positive and empowering aspect of your overall well-being. Remember, the choices you make in the grocery store have a lasting impact on your health, and with each shopping trip, you have the opportunity to nourish your body and make strides toward a healthier, more vibrant lifestyle.

✓ Tips for a Healthy Cart

Creating a healthy grocery cart is a foundational step in promoting a nutritious and balanced diet. This guide aims to provide practical and easy-to-understand tips for selecting wholesome foods, making informed choices, and optimizing your shopping experience.

1. Start with Fresh Produce:

The foundation of a healthy cart begins in the produce section. Fill a significant portion of your cart with a colorful array of fruits and vegetables.

- Why it matters:
    - Fruits and vegetables are rich in essential vitamins, minerals, fiber, and antioxidants.
    - A diverse range of colors indicates a variety of nutrients, contributing to overall health.

- Tips:
    - Choose a mix of leafy greens, vibrant berries, cruciferous vegetables, and seasonal options.

- Consider fresh, frozen, or canned options based on availability and convenience.

2. Prioritize Whole Grains:

Opt for whole grains to provide a nutritious foundation for your meals.

- Why it matters:
    - Whole grains offer complex carbohydrates, fiber, and various essential nutrients.
    - They contribute to sustained energy, digestive health, and a feeling of fullness.

- Tips:

- Choose whole grain options such as brown rice, quinoa, whole wheat bread, and oats.

- Read labels to ensure products are made with whole grains rather than refined grains.

3. Select Lean Proteins:

Incorporate lean protein sources to support muscle health and satiety.

- Why it matters:

- Proteins are essential for building and repairing tissues, supporting immune function, and maintaining a healthy weight.

- Lean proteins offer these benefits without excess saturated fats.

- Tips:

  - Choose options like skinless poultry, fish, lean cuts of meat, tofu, legumes, and low-fat dairy.

  - Consider plant-based protein sources for variety, such as beans, lentils, and edamame.

4. Include Healthy Fats:

Add sources of healthy fats to your cart for heart health and overall well-being.

- Why it matters:

  - Healthy fats play a crucial role in nutrient absorption, brain function, and cell structure.

  - They contribute to feelings of fullness and satisfaction.

- Tips:

   - Include avocados, nuts, seeds, and olive oil in your cart.

   - Choose fatty fish like salmon for omega-3 fatty acids.

5. Be Mindful in the Dairy Aisle:

Navigate the dairy aisle with mindfulness, selecting options that align with your health goals.

- Why it matters:

   - Dairy products provide essential calcium, vitamin D, and protein.

   - Opting for low-fat or non-fat varieties reduces saturated fat intake.

- Tips:

- Choose low-fat or non-fat milk, yogurt, and cheese.

- Consider dairy alternatives like almond or soy milk for lactose intolerance or dietary preferences.

6. Mindful Beverage Choices:

Pay attention to beverage choices to ensure they contribute to your overall health.

- Why it matters:

- Hydration is essential for bodily functions and overall well-being.

- Sugary beverages can contribute to excess calories and may have negative effects on health.

- Tips:

- Make water your primary hydrating choice.

- Limit sugary drinks, opting for unsweetened beverages or herbal teas.

- Be mindful of portion sizes, even for healthier options like fruit juices.

7. Choose Whole, Minimally Processed Foods:

Prioritize whole, minimally processed foods over highly processed alternatives.

- Why it matters:

- Whole foods retain more nutrients and are often lower in added sugars, salt, and unhealthy fats.

- Minimally processed options support overall health and well-being.

- Tips:

  - Opt for whole fruits instead of fruit juices or fruit-flavored snacks.

  - Choose whole grains over refined grains for higher nutritional content.

8. Read Labels Carefully:

Take the time to read and understand food labels for informed decision-making.

- Why it matters:

  - Labels provide information about serving sizes, nutritional content, and ingredient lists.

  - Understanding labels helps you avoid hidden sugars, excessive sodium, and artificial additives.

- Tips:

- Pay attention to serving sizes to avoid overconsumption.

- Look for products with recognizable, whole-food ingredients.

- Be wary of marketing claims and focus on nutritional content.

9. Limit Processed and Sugary Snacks:

Be selective with snack choices, opting for healthier alternatives.

- Why it matters:

- Excessive consumption of processed and sugary snacks can contribute to weight gain and health issues.

- Choosing nutrient-dense snacks supports overall nutrition.

- Tips:
  - Choose snacks like nuts, seeds, fresh fruit, or yogurt.
  - Be mindful of portion sizes and avoid mindless snacking.

10. Plan for Healthy Meals:

Consider your weekly meal plan as you fill your cart to ensure you have all the necessary ingredients.

- Why it matters:
  - Meal planning reduces food waste, saves time, and promotes healthier eating habits.
  - Having a plan helps you avoid last-minute, less-healthy choices.

- Tips:

  - Check your pantry and refrigerator before shopping to avoid buying duplicates.

  - Use your shopping list to guide purchases based on planned meals.

11. Be Wary of Sales and Promotions:

While sales and promotions can save you money, approach them with mindfulness.

- Why it matters:

  - Impulse purchases driven by sales may lead to less healthy choices.

  - Being mindful ensures your choices align with your health goals.

- Tips:

- Stick to your shopping list and only purchase items on sale if they align with your needs.

- Be cautious of bulk purchases for perishable items that may lead to food waste.

12. Don't Shop Hungry:

Shopping on an empty stomach can lead to impulsive, less healthy choices.

- Why it matters:

- Hunger can influence food choices, leading to the purchase of less nutritious items.

- Eating before shopping helps you make rational decisions and stick to your planned purchases.

- Tips:

- Eat a balanced meal or snack before heading to the store.

- Carry a water bottle to stay hydrated and curb hunger.

13. Prioritize Seasonal and Local Produce:

Incorporate seasonal and local produce when possible for freshness and sustainability.

- Why it matters:

- Seasonal produce is often fresher, more affordable, and supports local agriculture.

- Choosing local options reduces environmental impact and promotes community well-being.

- Tips:

  - Familiarize yourself with seasonal produce in your region.

  - Explore local farmers' markets for fresh and diverse options.

14. Be Open to Trying New Foods:

Embrace variety in your diet by being open to trying new and unfamiliar foods.

- Why it matters:

  - A diverse diet provides a broad spectrum of nutrients and supports overall health.

  - Trying new foods adds excitement and variety to your meals.

- Tips:

  - Explore different fruits, vegetables, grains, and ethnic cuisines.

  - Incorporate one or two new items into your cart each shopping trip.

15. Reflect on Your Choices:

Periodically reflect on your grocery shopping choices to refine and improve your approach.

- Why it matters:

  - Reflection enhances your ability to make informed choices in the future.

  - Assessing what worked well and what could be improved contributes to a continuous improvement mindset.

- Tips:

- Consider how your choices align with your health goals.

- Adjust your shopping list based on reflections and evolving needs.

Creating a healthy grocery cart is a proactive and empowering step toward supporting your overall well-being. By incorporating these tips into your shopping routine, you can transform your cart into a collection of nutrient-rich, flavorful foods that contribute to a balanced and satisfying diet. Remember, the choices you make in the grocery store have a lasting impact on your health, and with each shopping trip, you have the opportunity to nourish your body and cultivate a lifestyle that promotes vitality and wellness.

✓ Reading Labels Like a Pro

Reading food labels is a crucial skill that empowers you to make informed and healthy choices while navigating the aisles of the grocery store. This guide aims to demystify the process of reading labels, providing you with practical tips to decipher nutritional information, ingredient lists, and marketing claims.

• Understanding the Basics:

Before delving into the intricacies of food labels, let's start with the basics. Food labels are designed to provide consumers with information about the nutritional content of a product, helping you make informed decisions about what you eat. Key components of a food label include:

1. Serving Size:

- This indicates the recommended portion size for the product. All other information on the label is based on this serving size.

2. Calories:

- The number of calories per serving provides insight into the energy content of the food.

3. Nutrients:

- Essential nutrients are listed along with their quantity per serving. Common nutrients include fats, carbohydrates, protein, vitamins, and minerals.

4. % Daily Value (%DV):

- This percentage indicates how much a nutrient in a serving contributes to a daily diet based on a standard daily intake of 2,000 calories. It helps you assess the nutritional significance of a particular nutrient in the context of your overall diet.

Now, let's explore how to read labels effectively:

1. Start with the Serving Size:

Understanding the serving size is crucial because all other nutritional information on the label is based on it. Compare the serving size listed on the label to the amount you typically consume. If you eat more or less than the specified serving size, you'll need to adjust the nutrient values accordingly.

- Example:
  - If the serving size is 1 cup, but you typically eat 2 cups, you'll need to double the values for calories and nutrients.

2. Check the Calories:

Calories provide a measure of the energy content in a serving. Be mindful of the calorie count, especially if you're managing your weight or monitoring your energy intake.

- Example:

- If a serving has 200 calories, and you typically consume 2 servings, you'd be consuming 400 calories.

3. Assess Macronutrients:

Macronutrients include fats, carbohydrates, and protein. Understanding these components helps you balance your diet according to your nutritional needs.

- Fats:
  - Look for sources of healthy fats such as monounsaturated and polyunsaturated fats. Limit saturated and trans fats.
- Carbohydrates:
  - Choose products with complex carbohydrates (whole grains, fiber) over

refined carbohydrates. Be mindful of added sugars.
- Protein:
  - Opt for protein sources like lean meats, poultry, fish, beans, and legumes.

4. Pay Attention to % Daily Value (%DV):

The %DV is a quick reference guide to assess the nutritional significance of a specific nutrient based on a 2,000-calorie daily diet. Generally, a %DV of 5% or less is considered low, while 20% or more is considered high.

- Example:
  - If a product has 15% DV of fiber, it contributes significantly to your daily fiber needs.

5. Understand Ingredient Lists:

Ingredient lists provide insight into what a product contains. Ingredients are listed in descending order by weight, so the first few ingredients make up the majority of the product.

- Look for Whole Foods:
    - Choose products with whole, recognizable ingredients. This indicates a less processed and more nutritious option.

- Be Wary of Hidden Sugars and Additives:
    - Ingredients like high-fructose corn syrup, artificial sweeteners, and

preservatives may be hidden sources of unwanted additives.

6. Beware of Marketing Claims:

While labels may boast various health claims, it's essential to critically evaluate them. Phrases like "low-fat," "organic," or "natural" can be misleading.

- Example:
    - A "low-fat" product might compensate with added sugars or artificial additives for flavor.

7. Watch Out for Serving Size Tricks:

Manufacturers sometimes manipulate serving sizes to make products appear healthier than they are. Be aware of this tactic and assess your actual consumption.

- Example:

  - A small bag of chips might list a small serving size to make the calorie content seem lower than if you were to eat the entire bag.

8. Be Mindful of Allergens:

Food labels also provide information about common allergens like nuts, dairy, soy, and gluten. If you have allergies or intolerances, carefully review these sections of the label.

- Example:

- If you're allergic to nuts, check for potential cross-contamination or hidden sources of nuts in the ingredient list.

9. Consider Nutrient Density:

Nutrient-dense foods provide a high amount of essential nutrients relative to their calorie content. Aim to choose foods that offer substantial nutritional value per calorie.

- Example:

- Vegetables and fruits are nutrient-dense choices because they provide vitamins, minerals, and fiber with relatively few calories.

10. Look for Added Sugars:

Identifying added sugars is crucial, especially since many processed foods contain hidden sugars that contribute to excessive calorie intake.

- Example:
    - Ingredients like sucrose, high-fructose corn syrup, and agave syrup indicate added sugars.

11. Be Skeptical of Front-of-Package Claims:

Front-of-package claims are designed to catch your attention, but they may not tell the whole story. Flip the product and examine the nutrition label and ingredient list for a comprehensive view.

- Example:

  - A "heart-healthy" claim on the front might not consider other aspects like sodium content.

12. Compare Similar Products:

When choosing between similar products, compare their nutritional content, ingredient lists, and %DV to make the best choice for your health.

- Example:

  - Compare two brands of yogurt to see which one offers more protein, less sugar, or additional nutrients.

Putting It All Together:

Reading food labels like a pro involves a holistic understanding of serving sizes, calories, macronutrients, %DV, ingredient lists, and marketing claims. With this knowledge, you can make informed decisions that align with your health goals and preferences.

Example Scenario:

Imagine you're choosing between two breakfast cereals:

1. Cereal A:
    - Serving Size: 1 cup
    - Calories: 120 per serving
    - Total Fat: 2g (3% DV)
    - Sodium: 150mg (6% DV)
    - Total Carbohydrates: 24g (8% DV)
    - Dietary Fiber: 5g (20% DV)

- Sugars: 6g
- Protein: 3g

2. Cereal B:
  - Serving Size: 1 cup
  - Calories: 160 per serving
  - Total Fat: 4g (6% DV)
  - Sodium: 120mg (5% DV)
  - Total Carbohydrates: 30g (10% DV)
  - Dietary Fiber: 4g (16% DV)
  - Sugars: 8g
  - Protein: 2g

Analysis:

- Calories:

  - Cereal A has fewer calories per serving than Cereal B, making it a slightly lighter option.

- Fiber:

  - Cereal A has more fiber, contributing to better digestive health and increased satiety.

- Protein:

  - Cereal B has slightly less protein, so if protein intake is a priority, you might lean towards Cereal A

- Sugars:

  - Both cereals contain added sugars, but Cereal A has less, making it a better option if you're watching your sugar intake.

- Fat:

  - Cereal B has slightly more fat, but the type of fat is essential. If it contains healthy fats like nuts or seeds, this may be a favorable choice.

In this scenario, your decision might depend on your specific health goals. If you prioritize lower sugar and higher fiber content, Cereal A might be the preferred option.

Reading food labels like a pro is an invaluable skill for making informed and health-conscious choices. By understanding the basics, being aware of serving sizes, assessing macronutrients, scrutinizing ingredient lists, and being cautious of marketing claims, you can confidently navigate the grocery store aisles. Remember, the goal is to choose foods that align with your health goals, preferences, and overall well-being. Armed with this knowledge, you can approach food labels with confidence and make choices that contribute to a balanced and nutritious diet.

CHAPTER 4

EASY MEAL PLANNING

*E*asy meal planning is a foundational skill that can simplify your life, save you time, and contribute to a healthier, more balanced diet. This comprehensive guide will break down the process of meal planning into manageable steps, providing practical tips and strategies to make meal planning a seamless part of your routine. Whether you're a beginner or looking to enhance your existing meal planning skills, this guide aims to make the process easy, enjoyable, and effective.

• Understanding the Benefits of Meal Planning:

Meal planning offers a multitude of benefits, including:

1. Time Savings:
   - Planning meals in advance reduces the time spent deciding what to cook each day. It streamlines grocery shopping and preparation.

2. Healthier Choices:

- Thoughtful planning allows you to incorporate a variety of nutrient-dense foods, ensuring a balanced and healthful diet.

3. Cost-Efficiency:

- By creating a shopping list based on planned meals, you can avoid impulsive purchases and minimize food waste, leading to cost savings.

4. Reduced Stress:

- Knowing what you'll eat eliminates the stress of last-minute decisions. It adds structure to your daily routine and enhances overall well-being.

5. Variety and Creativity:

- Planning meals in advance encourages experimentation with new recipes and ingredients, adding variety and excitement to your meals.

• Getting Started with Meal Planning:

1. Assess Your Schedule:

Consider your weekly commitments, work hours, and any social events. This understanding helps tailor your meal plan to fit your schedule, ensuring that meals are realistic and achievable.

2. Define Your Goals:

Clearly outline your meal planning objectives. Whether it's weight management, saving time, or adopting a healthier diet, having specific goals guides your choices.

3. Create a Weekly Calendar:

Outline a weekly calendar, including breakfast, lunch, dinner, and snacks. This visual aid provides a clear overview of your meals for the week.

4. Take Inventory:

Check your pantry, refrigerator, and freezer to see what ingredients you already have. Incorporate these items into your meal plan to minimize waste and save money.

5. Consider Dietary Preferences and Restrictions:

Account for any dietary preferences or restrictions. Whether you're vegetarian, gluten-free, or have specific allergies, tailor your meals accordingly.

6. Gather Recipe Inspiration:

Collect recipe ideas from cookbooks, websites, or family favorites. Having a pool of recipes to draw from makes meal planning more enjoyable and varied.

The Basic Components of Meal Planning:

1. Plan Your Meals:

Start by deciding what meals you'll prepare for the week. Consider a mix of cuisines, cooking techniques, and a balance of protein, carbohydrates, and vegetables.

- Example:
  - Monday: Grilled chicken with quinoa and roasted vegetables.
  - Tuesday: Spaghetti Bolognese with a side salad.
  - Wednesday: Vegetarian stir-fry with tofu and brown rice.

2. Create a Shopping List:

Based on your planned meals, compile a comprehensive shopping list. Group items by category (produce, dairy, etc.) to streamline your shopping experience.

- Example:
  - Chicken breasts
  - Quinoa
  - Mixed vegetables
  - Ground beef
  - Whole wheat spaghetti
  - Salad greens
  - Tofu
  - Brown rice

3. Batch Cooking:

Consider batch cooking certain ingredients to use in multiple meals. For example, cook a batch of quinoa or roast a large tray of vegetables that can be incorporated into different dishes.

4. Mix and Match:

Create versatility within your plan. For instance, roast extra vegetables that can be used in salads, wraps, or alongside another main dish later in the week.

5. Embrace Simplicity:

Not every meal needs to be elaborate. Include simple recipes that require minimal ingredients and preparation for busier days.

6. Use Leftovers Creatively:

Plan meals that can easily transform into the next day's lunch or dinner. For example, turn grilled chicken from dinner into a chicken salad for lunch.

Tips for Practical Meal Planning:

1. Theme Nights:

Assign themes to different days of the week to simplify decision-making. For example, "Meatless Monday," "Taco Tuesday," or "Stir-Fry Friday."

2. Prep Ingredients in Advance:

Chop vegetables, marinate proteins, or prepare grains in advance. Having ingredients ready expedites the cooking process during busy weekdays.

3. Be Flexible:

Life is unpredictable, so allow for flexibility in your meal plan. Have a few backup options or consider designated "leftover nights.

4. Involve the Family:

Engage family members in the meal planning process. Encourage input and consider preferences to make meals enjoyable for everyone.

5. Plan for Convenience:

Incorporate convenience items like pre-cut vegetables or pre-cooked grains to streamline preparation, especially on hectic days.

6. Utilize Technology:

Explore meal planning apps or websites that offer recipes, generate shopping lists, and provide nutritional information.

7. Plan for Variety:

Ensure variety in your meals to prevent monotony. Rotate proteins, grains, and vegetables to keep your meals exciting and satisfying.

Sample Meal Plan:

Monday:
- Breakfast: Greek yogurt with berries and granola.
- Lunch: Quinoa salad with mixed vegetables and feta cheese.

- Dinner: Baked salmon with sweet potato and steamed broccoli.

Tuesday:
- Breakfast: Oatmeal with sliced banana and almond butter.
- Lunch: Whole grain wrap with turkey, lettuce, and tomato.
- Dinner: Vegetarian stir-fry with tofu and brown rice.

Wednesday:
- Breakfast: Smoothie with spinach, banana, and protein powder.
- Lunch: Chickpea salad with cucumber, cherry tomatoes, and feta.
- Dinner: Spaghetti Bolognese with a side salad.

Thursday:

- Breakfast: Whole grain toast with avocado and poached egg.
- Lunch: Lentil soup with whole grain crackers.
- Dinner: Grilled chicken with quinoa and roasted vegetables.

Friday:
- Breakfast: Cottage cheese with pineapple and a sprinkle of chia seeds.
- Lunch: Caesar salad with grilled chicken.
- Dinner: Homemade pizza with a variety of vegetable toppings.

• Troubleshooting Common Challenges:

1. Lack of Inspiration:

If you find yourself in a culinary rut, explore new recipes, cuisines, or cooking techniques. Engage with online communities for inspiration.

2. Time Constraints:

Choose recipes with shorter preparation and cooking times on busier days. Utilize batch cooking and consider make-ahead options.

3. Overcommitting:

Be realistic about the time you have available for cooking. If your schedule is hectic, opt for simpler recipes or designate certain days for leftovers.

4. Food Preferences:

If a family member has specific food preferences, incorporate their favorite meals into the plan. Finding a balance ensures everyone is satisfied.

5. Inadequate Planning:

Avoid last-minute decisions by consistently setting aside time each week for meal planning. Make it a routine to enhance efficiency.

In conclusion, Meal planning is a dynamic and flexible process that adapts to your lifestyle and preferences. By breaking down the steps, incorporating practical tips, and embracing a variety of recipes, you can make meal planning an enjoyable and sustainable practice. .

✓ Creating Diabetes-Friendly Menus

Creating diabetes-friendly menus involves thoughtful planning and a focus on balanced, nutritious meals. This guide breaks down the process into simple steps, offering practical tips to help you design menus that align with diabetes management. Whether you're managing your own diabetes or preparing meals for someone else, understanding the basics of a diabetes-friendly menu empowers you to make informed and health-conscious choices.

• Understanding Diabetes-Friendly Nutrition:

1. Emphasize Whole, Unprocessed Foods:

Incorporate whole, unprocessed foods into your meals. These include fruits, vegetables, lean proteins, whole grains, and healthy fats. Whole foods provide essential nutrients, fiber, and a slower release of glucose into the bloodstream.

- Example:
  - Instead of white rice, opt for brown rice or quinoa.
  - Choose fresh fruits instead of fruit juices or sugary snacks.

2. Balance Carbohydrates:

Carbohydrates impact blood sugar levels, so it's essential to balance their intake. Choose complex carbohydrates with a lower glycemic index to help manage blood sugar.

- Example:
    - Include whole grains like oats, barley, or whole wheat bread.
    - Pair carbohydrates with protein and healthy fats to slow the absorption of sugar.

3. Portion Control:

Managing portion sizes is crucial for diabetes management. Pay attention to portion control to avoid spikes in blood sugar levels.

- Example:

  - Use smaller plates to help control portion sizes.

  - Be mindful of serving sizes for grains, proteins, and high-carb vegetables.

4. Prioritize Lean Proteins:

Incorporate lean protein sources, such as poultry, fish, tofu, and legumes. Protein helps stabilize blood sugar levels and promotes satiety.

- Example:

  - Choose skinless poultry or fish for main dishes.

  - Include plant-based proteins like beans or lentils in your meals.

5. Opt for Healthy Fats:

Include sources of healthy fats in your menu, such as avocados, nuts, seeds, and olive oil. Healthy fats contribute to overall well-being and help manage blood sugar.

- Example:
  - Use olive oil for cooking and as a dressing for salads.
  - Include a small serving of nuts or seeds as a snack.

6. Incorporate Fiber-Rich Foods:

Fiber aids in digestion and helps regulate blood sugar levels. Include a variety of fiber-rich foods in your menu, such as fruits, vegetables, whole grains, and legumes.

- Example:
    - Snack on raw vegetables with hummus.
    - Choose high-fiber cereals or add chia seeds to your yogurt.

7. Limit Added Sugars:

Minimize the consumption of added sugars in your menu. Choose naturally sweet foods and use alternatives like stevia or monk fruit when necessary.

- Example:
    - Opt for plain yogurt and add fresh fruit for sweetness.

- Limit sugary beverages and choose water or unsweetened alternatives.

• Creating Balanced Diabetes-Friendly Menus:

1. Plan Meals in Advance:

Develop a weekly meal plan to ensure balanced and varied nutrition. Consider breakfast, lunch, dinner, and snacks to maintain consistent energy levels throughout the day.

- Example:

  - Plan a breakfast with a mix of protein (e.g., eggs), complex carbohydrates (e.g., whole grain toast), and healthy fats (e.g., avocado).

2. Diversify Your Protein Sources:

Incorporate a variety of protein sources to enhance the nutritional profile of your meals. This ensures you receive a range of essential amino acids.

- Example:
  - Include fish, poultry, tofu, beans, and lean meats throughout the week.

3. Build Colorful, Nutrient-Rich Plates:

Create visually appealing plates by including a variety of colorful fruits and vegetables. Different colors often indicate a diverse range of nutrients.

- Example:

- Add a mix of colorful vegetables to your stir-fry or salad.
- Include berries or citrus fruits for a vibrant and nutritious dessert.

4. Consider Meal Timing:

Pay attention to the timing of your meals and snacks. Spreading meals throughout the day helps regulate blood sugar levels and prevents extreme fluctuations.

- Example:
  - Include a mid-morning or afternoon snack to maintain steady energy levels.
  - Avoid long periods without food to prevent overeating during main meals.

5. Prepare Snacks Mindfully:

Choose diabetes-friendly snacks that provide nutritional benefits without causing rapid spikes in blood sugar. Pairing a carbohydrate with protein or healthy fats can be a smart choice.

- Example:
   - Snack on a small apple with a handful of almonds.
   - Greek yogurt with berries makes for a satisfying and balanced snack.

6. Hydration Matters:

Stay hydrated with water and other non-caloric beverages. Limit sugary drinks and be mindful of the impact of caffeine on blood sugar levels.

- Example:

  - Infuse water with citrus slices or cucumber for added flavor.

  - Choose herbal teas or black coffee without added sugars.

7. Experiment with Herbs and Spices:

Enhance the flavor of your meals with herbs and spices instead of relying on excessive salt or sugar. Experimenting with different seasonings adds variety to your menu.

- Example:

  - Use herbs like basil, thyme, or rosemary for seasoning.

  - Spice up dishes with cinnamon or cumin for added depth.

8. Listen to Your Body:

Pay attention to your body's hunger and fullness cues. Eat mindfully and savor each bite to avoid overeating.

- Example:
  - Pause between bites and enjoy the flavors of your meal.
    - Stop eating when you feel comfortably satisfied.

• Sample Diabetes-Friendly Menu:

Day 1:

Breakfast:
- Scrambled eggs with spinach and whole grain toast.

Lunch:
- Grilled chicken salad with mixed greens, cherry tomatoes, and balsamic vinaigrette.

Dinner:
- Baked salmon with quinoa and steamed broccoli.

Snack:
- Greek yogurt with a sprinkle of chia seeds.

Day 2:

Breakfast:
- Overnight oats with almond milk, sliced strawberries, and a dollop of almond butter.

Lunch:
- Whole grain wrap with turkey, avocado, lettuce, and tomato.

Dinner:
- Vegetarian stir-fry with tofu, broccoli, bell peppers, and brown rice.

Snack:
- Carrot sticks with hummus.

Day 3:

Breakfast:
- Smoothie with kale, banana, Greek yogurt, and a handful of blueberries.

Lunch:
- Lentil soup with a side of whole grain crackers.

Dinner:
- Grilled shrimp with quinoa and roasted asparagus.

Snack:
- Handful of mixed nuts.

Creating diabetes-friendly menus is about making informed choices that prioritize balanced nutrition and support blood sugar management. By focusing on whole, unprocessed foods, balancing macronutrients, and planning meals in advance, you can design menus that are not only delicious but also contribute to overall well-being.

✓ **Cooking In Batches For Convenience**

Cooking in batches is a practical and time-efficient approach that can simplify your meal preparation, save you time, and contribute to a more convenient and stress-free cooking experience. This guide will break down the process of cooking in batches into simple steps, providing practical tips and strategies to help you incorporate batch cooking into your routine.

• Understanding the Benefits of Batch Cooking:

1. Time Efficiency:

Batch cooking allows you to prepare multiple servings of a dish at once, reducing the time spent in the kitchen on a daily basis. This is particularly beneficial for individuals with busy schedules.

2. Cost Savings:

Buying ingredients in larger quantities for batch cooking can be cost-effective. You can take advantage of sales, discounts, and bulk purchases, ultimately saving money in the long run.

3. Minimizing Food Waste:

Batch cooking helps minimize food waste by allowing you to use ingredients efficiently. You can buy in bulk, use perishable items before they go bad, and repurpose leftovers creatively.

4. Consistent Nutrition:

By planning and cooking meals in batches, you have better control over the nutritional content of your meals. This consistency can be particularly important if you're managing specific dietary requirements or health goals.

5. Convenient Meal Planning:

Having pre-cooked meals on hand simplifies meal planning. You can mix and match components to create varied and balanced meals throughout the week without starting from scratch each time.

Getting Started with Batch Cooking:

1. Plan Your Menu:

Start by planning a menu for the week. Choose recipes that are suitable for batch cooking and can be easily stored or frozen. Consider meals that use similar ingredients to maximize efficiency.

- Example:
  - If you plan to cook grilled chicken for one meal, consider incorporating it into salads, wraps, or bowls for subsequent meals.

2. Choose Freezer-Friendly Recipes:

Opt for recipes that freeze well. Not all dishes maintain their quality after freezing, so select options that won't compromise taste and texture upon reheating.

- Example:

  - Soups, stews, casseroles, and certain types of pasta dishes often freeze and reheat successfully.

3. Invest in Quality Storage Containers:

Having reliable storage containers is crucial for batch cooking. Choose containers that are freezer-safe, airtight, and appropriately sized for single servings or family portions.

- Example:

  - Invest in reusable glass or plastic containers with secure lids.

- Consider using freezer bags for items like soups or sauces that can be laid flat for efficient storage.

4. Create a Batch Cooking Schedule:

Designate specific days for batch cooking to fit into your weekly routine. This could be on weekends when you have more time or a weekday evening when you can prepare meals for the upcoming days.

- Example:
    - Sunday: Batch cook proteins (chicken, beef, etc.).
    - Monday: Prepare grains (rice, quinoa, etc.) and chop vegetables.
  - Wednesday: Cook sauces or stews.

5. Stock Your Pantry:

Keep essential pantry items on hand for batch cooking. This includes staples like grains, canned beans, and tomatoes, as well as a variety of herbs and spices to add flavor to your dishes.

- Example:
    - Keep a selection of dried herbs, spices, olive oil, and vinegar for seasoning.
    - Maintain a well-stocked pantry of canned goods for quick additions to recipes.

6. Utilize Kitchen Appliances:

Leverage kitchen appliances to make batch cooking more efficient. Slow cookers, Instant Pots, and large baking sheets can be valuable tools for preparing larger quantities of food.

- Example:
  - Use an Instant Pot to cook large batches of chili or soup.
  - Roast vegetables on a baking sheet for easy meal additions.

Batch Cooking Techniques:

1. Pre-Cook Proteins:

Prepare proteins in advance and use them as versatile ingredients throughout the week. Cooked proteins can be added to salads, wraps, sandwiches, or served with a variety of side dishes.

- Example:

 - Grill or roast chicken breasts for use in multiple meals.

 - Cook ground turkey or beef to add to pasta dishes or tacos.

2. Cook Grains in Batches:

Cooking grains in larger quantities saves time and provides a foundation for various meals. Grains like rice, quinoa, or couscous can be portioned and refrigerated or frozen.

- Example:

 - Cook a batch of brown rice to use in stir-fries, burrito bowls, or alongside proteins.

3. Prepare Saucy Dishes:

Prepare saucy dishes like casseroles, curries, or stews in larger quantities. These dishes often improve in flavor when reheated.

- Example:
  - Make a hearty vegetable stew that can be portioned for several meals.
  - Cook a large batch of tomato sauce for pasta or pizza.

4. Freeze Individual Portions:

After cooking in batches, portion meals into individual servings before freezing. This makes it easy to thaw only what you need, reducing the risk of food going to waste.

- Example:

  - Freeze individual servings of soup, chili, or lasagna for quick and convenient meals.

5. Create Meal Components:

Prepare components that can be combined in different ways. For example, roasted vegetables, cooked proteins, and grains can be mixed and matched for various meals.

- Example:

  - Roast a variety of vegetables to use in salads, wraps, or as side dishes.
  - Cook a large batch of quinoa to serve as a base for different meals.

Tips for Successful Batch Cooking:

1. Label Containers:

Clearly label containers with the date of preparation and contents. This ensures you can easily identify items in your freezer and maintain an organized system.

2. Rotate Your Stock:

When adding new batch-cooked items to the freezer, rotate older items to the front. This helps ensure that older meals are used before they reach their limit for quality.

3. Keep a Variety:

Create a variety of dishes to prevent monotony. This ensures that you look forward to your meals and helps you maintain a balanced diet.

4. Consider Thawing Methods:

Plan ahead for thawing. Some items may need to be transferred from the freezer to the refrigerator a day before use, while others can be thawed more quickly in the microwave.

5. Tailor to Your Needs:

Adapt batch cooking to your specific dietary needs and preferences. Whether you follow a specific diet or have particular taste preferences, tailor your batch-cooked meals accordingly.

• Sample Batch Cooking Menu:

Batch Cooking Day:

Proteins:
- Grill or roast chicken breasts.
- Cook ground turkey with herbs and spices.
- Prepare a batch of lentils in the Instant Pot.

Grains:
- Cook a large batch of quinoa.
- Prepare brown rice in the rice cooker.

Saucy Dishes:
- Make a vegetable and chickpea curry.
- Prepare a hearty vegetable and bean stew.

Components:
- Roast a mix of vegetables (bell peppers, zucchini, cherry tomatoes).
- Cook a large batch of tomato sauce.

Throughout the Week:

Meal 1:
- Grilled chicken with quinoa and roasted vegetables.

Meal 2:
- Lentil salad with mixed greens and vinaigrette.

Meal 3:
- Spaghetti with tomato sauce and ground turkey.

Meal 4:
- Chickpea curry with brown rice.

Snack:
- Greek yogurt with a drizzle of honey and a handful of berries.

In essence, Batch cooking is a valuable skill that can transform your approach to meal preparation. By planning, organizing, and utilizing time-saving techniques, you can enjoy the benefits of efficiency, cost savings, and reduced food waste. Whether you're cooking for yourself, your family, or simply looking to make your daily routine more manageable, batch cooking is a practical and accessible solution. With the right mindset and a bit of preparation, you can integrate batch cooking into your lifestyle and experience the convenience of having delicious, homemade meals at your fingertips.

CHAPTER 5

DELICIOUS CARB ALTERNATIVES

Exploring Delicious Carb Alternatives

• Cauliflower Creations

In the world of carb alternatives, cauliflower emerges as a versatile hero. Let's dive into two scrumptious recipes that reimagine familiar favorites.

Recipe 1: Cauliflower Pizza Crust

Ingredients:
- Cauliflower rice
- Eggs
- Parmesan cheese
- Italian seasoning

Instructions:
1. Prepare Cauliflower Rice: Grate cauliflower into a fine, rice-like consistency.
2. Cook Cauliflower: Steam or microwave cauliflower rice until tender.
3. Create Dough: Mix cauliflower rice with beaten eggs, Parmesan cheese, and Italian seasoning.
4. Shape Crust: Press the mixture into a thin, round shape on a baking sheet.
5. Bake: Watch as the crust transforms into a golden masterpiece.

Result: A low-carb pizza crust ready for your favorite toppings.

Recipe 2: Eggplant Lasagna Roll-Ups

Ingredients:
- Sliced eggplant
- Ricotta cheese
- Spinach
- Marinara sauce
- Mozzarella cheese

Instructions:
1. Prepare Eggplant: Grill or bake sliced eggplant until pliable.
2. Make Filling: Mix ricotta cheese with chopped spinach.
3. Roll and Fill: Spread ricotta mixture on each eggplant slice and roll up.

4. Bake: Place the rolls in a baking dish, cover with marinara sauce and mozzarella cheese, and bake until bubbly.

Result: A carb-conscious, flavorful twist on traditional lasagna.

• Beyond the Ordinary

Recipe 3: Cauliflower Gnocchi with Pesto Sauce

Ingredients:
- Cauliflower gnocchi
- Homemade or store-bought pesto sauce
- Cherry tomatoes
- Grated Parmesan cheese

Instructions:

1. Cook Gnocchi: Boil or sauté cauliflower gnocchi according to package instructions.

2. Toss with Pesto: Coat cooked gnocchi with pesto sauce.

3. Add Toppings: Mix in halved cherry tomatoes and sprinkle with grated Parmesan cheese.

Result: A light and tasty alternative to traditional potato gnocchi.

Recipe 4: Sweet Potato Toast with Avocado and Poached Egg

Ingredients:
- Sweet potato slices
- Ripe avocado
- Eggs

- Salt, pepper, and chili flakes

Instructions:

1. Toast Sweet Potato: Toast sweet potato slices until tender.

2. Prepare Avocado: Mash ripe avocado and spread it over the sweet potato toast.

3. Add Egg: Poach eggs and place them on top of the avocado.

4. Season: Sprinkle with salt, pepper, and chili flakes.

Result: A nutrient-packed breakfast or snack with a medley of flavors.

• Lighter Bites

Recipe 5: Lettuce Wrap Tacos

Ingredients:
- Large lettuce leaves
- Seasoned ground turkey or beef
- Salsa, guacamole, shredded cheese

Instructions:
1. Cook Meat: Brown seasoned ground turkey or beef in a pan.
2. Wrap and Fill: Spoon the meat into lettuce leaves.
3. Add Toppings: Top with salsa, guacamole, and shredded cheese.

Result: A carb-free twist on classic tacos, perfect for a light lunch or dinner.

These delicious carb alternatives provide a delightful array of options if you're seeking to reduce carb intake or infuse creativity into your meals.

✓ Tasty Substitutes to Explore

• Unveiling Flavorful Alternatives

Embarking on a journey of culinary exploration introduces us to a world of tasty substitutes that promise to elevate our dishes. These alternatives not only cater to various dietary preferences but also infuse a delightful diversity of flavors into our meals. Join us as we uncover the art of tasteful substitutions.

Substitute 1: Cauliflower Mash with Garlic and Herbs

Ingredients:
- Cauliflower
- Garlic cloves

- Fresh herbs (rosemary, thyme)
- Butter or olive oil

Instructions:

1. Steam or Boil Cauliflower: Cook cauliflower until tender.

2. Mash with Flavor: Mash cauliflower with roasted garlic, fresh herbs, and a touch of butter or olive oil.

3. Serve: Enjoy as a flavorful alternative to traditional mashed potatoes.

Result: A velvety and aromatic side dish that transforms the humble cauliflower into a culinary masterpiece.

Substitute 2: Grilled Zucchini Ribbons with Pesto

Ingredients:

- Zucchini
- Homemade or store-bought pesto sauce
- Cherry tomatoes
- Pine nuts

Instructions:

1. Create Zucchini Ribbons: Use a vegetable peeler to create thin zucchini ribbons.

2. Grill or Sauté: Cook the zucchini ribbons until slightly tender.

3. Toss with Pesto: Coat the ribbons in pesto sauce, add halved cherry tomatoes, and sprinkle with pine nuts.

Result: A light and refreshing alternative to pasta, bursting with vibrant colors and flavors.

Substitute 3: Cauliflower Fried Rice with Mixed Vegetables

Ingredients:
- Cauliflower rice
- Mixed vegetables (peas, carrots, corn)
- Soy sauce
- Scrambled eggs

Instructions:
1. Prepare Cauliflower Rice: Grate cauliflower into rice-sized pieces.
2. Stir-Fry Vegetables: Sauté mixed vegetables in a pan.
3. Combine Ingredients: Mix cauliflower rice with stir-fried vegetables and scrambled eggs.
4. Season: Drizzle with soy sauce and toss until well combined.

Result: A low-carb and savory alternative to traditional fried rice, packed with wholesome goodness.

Substitute 4: Spiralized Zucchini Noodles with Avocado Pesto**

Ingredients:
- Zucchini noodles
- Ripe avocados
- Fresh basil
- Garlic
- Lemon juice

Instructions:
1. Create Zucchini Noodles: Spiralize zucchini into noodle-like strands.
2. Blend Avocado Pesto: Combine ripe avocados, fresh basil, garlic, and lemon juice in a blender.

3. Toss Together: Mix zucchini noodles with the creamy avocado pesto.

Result: A luscious and guilt-free alternative to traditional pasta, offering a creamy and green twist.

Substitute 5: Cauliflower Steak with Chimichurri Sauce

Ingredients:
- Thick cauliflower slices
- Chimichurri sauce (parsley, garlic, olive oil, red wine vinegar)

Instructions:
1. Slice Cauliflower Steaks: Cut cauliflower into thick slices to resemble steaks.

2. Grill or Roast: Cook cauliflower steaks until golden and slightly crispy.
3. Dress with Chimichurri: Drizzle chimichurri sauce over the cauliflower steaks before serving.

Result: A hearty and savory alternative to meat, with the vibrant flavors of chimichurri.

Substitute 6: Sweet Potato Toast with Nut Butter and Berries

Ingredients:
- Sweet potato slices
- Nut butter (almond, peanut, or cashew)
- Fresh berries

Instructions:

1. Toast Sweet Potato: Toast sweet potato slices until golden and tender.
2. Spread Nut Butter: Smear your favorite nut butter on the sweet potato slices.
3. Top with Berries: Garnish with a handful of fresh berries.

Result: A nutrient-packed and sweet alternative to traditional toast, perfect for a satisfying breakfast or snack.

Dive into the realm of tasty substitutes, where ordinary ingredients transform into extraordinary culinary creations. These alternatives not only cater to various dietary needs but also promise to tantalize your taste buds with an array of textures and flavors.

✓ Adding Excitement to Your Plate

• Understanding the Essence of Culinary Excitement

In the world of culinary delights, the concept of adding excitement to your plate goes beyond the ordinary. It's a journey that involves a harmonious blend of flavors, textures, and visual appeal. Let's unravel the essence of culinary excitement and discover how you can elevate your meals to a new level of enjoyment.

1. Flavor Variety:
   - Description: Culinary excitement begins with a spectrum of flavors. Incorporate sweet, savory, sour, bitter, and umami elements into your dishes to

create a well-balanced and dynamic taste experience.

- Tip: Experiment with different herbs, spices, and condiments to discover unique flavor combinations.

2. Textural Contrast:

- Description: Explore a range of textures to keep your palate engaged. Combine crispy with creamy, smooth with crunchy, and tender with chewy for a satisfying and interesting mouthfeel.

- Tip: Incorporate ingredients like nuts, seeds, or croutons to add crunchiness to salads or creamy sauces to complement grilled proteins.

3. Visual Appeal:

- Description: The presentation of a dish significantly impacts your dining experience. Play with colors, shapes, and arrangement to make your plate visually appealing. A visually enticing meal is often more enjoyable.

- Tip: Use vibrant and contrasting colors, garnishes, and edible flowers to enhance the visual appeal of your dishes.

4. Culinary Techniques:

- Description: Experiment with different cooking methods and techniques to enhance the depth of flavors. Grilling, roasting, sautéing, and marinating can elevate ingredients and bring out their unique qualities.

- Tip: Learn and master various cooking techniques to add layers of complexity to your dishes.

5. Simple Ways to Add Excitement:

1. Global Flavors Exploration:

- Description: Take a culinary journey by exploring global flavors. Incorporate spices, herbs, and condiments from various cuisines to add depth and complexity to your dishes.

- Tip: Research and try recipes from different cultures to broaden your flavor palate.

2. Colorful Veggie Bowls:

- Description: Create vibrant bowls filled with an array of colorful vegetables. Mix and match different veggies to add visual appeal and nutritional variety to your meals.

- Tip: Include a variety of vegetables in different colors, such as bell peppers, cherry tomatoes, and leafy greens.

3. Fresh Herb Infusion:
    - Description: Elevate your dishes with the freshness of herbs. Experiment with basil, cilantro, mint, or dill to add aromatic accents to salads, soups, and main courses.
    - Tip: Grow a small herb garden at home for a convenient and fresh supply of herbs.

4. Citrus Zest and Juices:
    - Description: Citrus fruits like lemons, limes, and oranges can bring a burst of brightness to your plate. Use zest and juices to enhance marinades, dressings, and desserts.

- Tip: Invest in a citrus zester to easily add citrus zest to your dishes.

5. Homemade Sauces and Condiments:
- Description: Create your own sauces and condiments to personalize flavors. Try making a garlic aioli, chimichurri, or tzatziki to add a gourmet touch to your meals.
- Tip: Experiment with different ingredients to create signature sauces that complement your favorite dishes.

• Guidelines for Culinary Excitement:

1. Balance is Key:
- Tip: While experimenting with flavors and textures, maintain a balance to ensure that no single element

overwhelms the dish. Aim for harmony in taste and presentation.

2. Season Thoughtfully:
   - Tip: Season dishes at various stages of cooking to layer flavors. Taste as you go and adjust seasoning to achieve a well-balanced and nuanced taste.

3. Embrace Seasonal Ingredients:
   - Tip: Incorporate seasonal produce to take advantage of peak freshness and flavor. Seasonal ingredients often add natural excitement to your plate.

4. Play with Temperature Contrasts:
   - Tip: Explore temperature contrasts in your meals. Serve warm dishes with cool or room-temperature

accompaniments to create a dynamic eating experience.

5. Mindful Plating:

- Tip: Pay attention to how you plate your dishes. Consider the arrangement, use of negative space, and the visual flow to make each dish visually appealing.

6. Family and Friends Involvement:

- Tip: Make the process of adding excitement to your plate a social one. Involve family or friends in the preparation, creating memorable experiences together.

7. Seasonal Menus and Themes:

- Tip: Plan seasonal menus or themed dinners to add an element of excitement. This can make meal planning more enjoyable and introduce variety to your routine.

8. Interactive Dining Experiences:
   - Tip: Consider interactive dining experiences, such as DIY taco bars or build-your-own pizza nights. This allows everyone to customize their plate according to their preferences.

9. Flavorful Garnishes:
   - Tip: Elevate your dishes with flavorful garnishes. Fresh herbs, citrus zest, or a drizzle of infused oil can enhance both taste and presentation.

10. Cooking Classes and Workshops:
    - Tip: Attend cooking classes or workshops to learn new techniques and

flavor combinations. Bringing fresh inspiration to your kitchen can add excitement to your cooking routine.

• Mouthwatering Recipes to Inspire Culinary Excitement:

1. Mango Avocado Salsa
2. Balsamic Strawberry Bruschetta
3. Spicy Honey Glazed Shrimp Skewers
4. Caprese Salad with a Twist
5. Grilled Pineapple Dessert Tacos
6. Lemon Herb Infused Quinoa Salad
7. Teriyaki Glazed Cauliflower Bites
8. Minty Watermelon Salad
9. Sesame Ginger Infused Stir-Fry
10. Dark Chocolate Dipped Citrus Slices

Adding excitement to your plate is a journey of culinary exploration, creativity, and a celebration of diverse flavors. By incorporating global influences, experimenting with fresh ingredients, and embracing various culinary techniques, you can turn every meal into a delightful experience. Whether you're a seasoned chef or just starting in the kitchen, infusing excitement into your plate is a simple yet rewarding endeavor. So, don your apron, gather your ingredients, and embark on a flavorful adventure that will not only tantalize your taste buds but also bring joy to your dining table. Cheers to savoring the excitement in every bite.

CHAPTER 6

EATING MINDFULLY FOR BLOOD SUGAR CONTROL

Let's explore the practice of eating mindfully for sugar control, emphasizing awareness, moderation, and thoughtful choices.

Eating Mindfully for Blood Sugar Control

• Nourishing Your Body with Awareness

In the realm of diabetes management, cultivating mindfulness around your dietary choices becomes a powerful tool for maintaining stable blood sugar levels. Let's delve into the principles of mindful eating and how they can contribute to better blood sugar control.

• Understanding Mindful Eating:
   - Description: Mindful eating is a practice that involves paying full attention to the sensory experience of eating. It promotes a heightened

awareness of taste, texture, and the act of consuming food.

- Tip: Begin each meal with a moment of gratitude for the nourishment your meal provides.

• Key Principles of Mindful Eating:

1. Eat with Intention:
- Tip: Set a clear intention for your meal. Consider the nutritional value and how the food will support your well-being.

2. Savor Each Bite:
- Tip: Take your time to chew and savor each bite. This not only aids digestion but also allows you to fully enjoy the flavors.

3. Be Present at Meals:

   - Tip: Minimize distractions during meals. Turn off electronic devices and focus on the act of eating without multitasking.

4. Listen to Hunger and Fullness Cues:

   - Tip: Tune in to your body's hunger and fullness signals. Eat when hungry, stop when satisfied, and avoid overeating.

5. Choose Nutrient-Dense Foods:

   - Tip: Prioritize nutrient-dense foods such as vegetables, lean proteins, and whole grains. These choices contribute to overall health and stable blood sugar.

6. Practice Portion Control:

- Tip: Be mindful of portion sizes. Use smaller plates to help regulate serving sizes and prevent overconsumption.

7. Mindful Snacking:
   - Tip: Snack with intention. Choose snacks that combine protein, fiber, and healthy fats to provide sustained energy and prevent blood sugar spikes.

8. Stay Hydrated:
   - Tip: Drink water throughout the day. Staying hydrated supports overall health and can help prevent overeating.

• Mindful Eating and Blood Sugar Control:

1. Understanding Glycemic Index:

- Description: The glycemic index (GI) measures how quickly a food raises blood sugar. Choose low-GI foods to promote gradual blood sugar increases.

- Tip: Include whole grains, legumes, and non-starchy vegetables in your diet for stable blood sugar levels.

2. Balancing Macronutrients:

- Description: Aim for a balanced mix of carbohydrates, proteins, and fats in each meal. This combination helps regulate blood sugar and provides sustained energy.

- Tip: Include lean proteins like poultry, fish, tofu, and healthy fats from sources like avocados and nuts.

3. Fiber-Rich Choices:

- Description: Fiber slows down the digestion and absorption of carbohydrates, promoting stable blood sugar levels.

- Tip: Incorporate fiber-rich foods such as fruits, vegetables, whole grains, and legumes into your meals.

• Mindfulness in Meal Planning:

1. Pre-Planning and Grocery Shopping:

- Tip: Plan your meals ahead of time and create a shopping list. This minimizes impulse purchases and ensures you have balanced ingredients on hand.

2. Reading Food Labels:

- Tip: Pay attention to food labels for information on carbohydrates, fiber, and added sugars. This empowers you to make informed choices.

3. Cooking with Consciousness:
   - Tip: Engage in the cooking process mindfully. Experiment with herbs and spices to enhance flavor without relying on excessive salt or sugar.

4. Mindful Dining Out:
   - Tip: When dining out, review the menu thoughtfully. Choose options that align with your dietary preferences and include a balance of nutrients.

• Mindfulness Beyond Meals:
1. Stress Management:
   - Description: Chronic stress can impact blood sugar levels. Incorporate stress-reducing activities such as

meditation, deep breathing, or hobbies into your routine.

- Tip: Prioritize self-care to promote overall well-being.

2. Regular Physical Activity:

- Description: Exercise helps regulate blood sugar levels. Include regular physical activity in your routine, such as brisk walking, cycling, or strength training.

- Tip: Find activities you enjoy to make exercise a sustainable part of your lifestyle.

Eating mindfully for blood sugar control is a holistic approach that encompasses awareness, thoughtful choices, and a harmonious relationship with food. By embracing the principles of mindful eating, you empower yourself to make informed decisions that support not only stable blood sugar levels but also overall well-being. Remember, each bite is an opportunity to nourish your body and savor the experience of enjoying wholesome and delicious food.

✓ Listening to Your Hunger and Fullness

• Tuning In to Your Body's Signals

In the journey of mindful eating, paying attention to your body's cues of hunger and fullness is a pivotal practice. Let's delve into the principles of listening to your body, fostering a more intuitive and nourishing approach to meals.

• Understanding Hunger and Fullness:

   - Description: Hunger and fullness are natural signals that indicate when to eat and when to stop. Tuning into these cues allows you to respond to your body's needs with awareness.

   - Tip: Start each meal by assessing your current hunger level on a scale from 1 to 10, with 1 being extremely hungry and 10 being overly full.

• Key Principles of Listening to Your Body:

1. Eat When Hungry:

   - Tip: Begin a meal when you feel genuine hunger. This ensures that you are eating to satisfy a physiological need rather than an emotional one.

2. Mindful Eating Practices:

- Tip: Engage in mindful practices such as deep breathing or a moment of gratitude before eating. This sets a positive tone for the meal and enhances your connection with the eating experience.

3. Slow Down:

- Tip: Eat at a moderate pace. Slow down to allow your body's satiety signals to catch up with your food intake.

4. Assess Fullness During Meals:

- Tip: Pause mid-meal to assess your fullness level. Check in with yourself and consider whether you're satisfied or if you're eating out of habit.

5. Hydrate Mindfully:

- Tip: Drink water throughout the meal, but avoid excessive drinking right before or during meals. Hydration is important, but too much liquid can impact your ability to recognize fullness.

6. Embrace Mindful Portion Control:

- Tip: Serve reasonable portions and allow yourself to have seconds if you're still genuinely hungry. Avoid feeling obligated to finish everything on your plate.

• Mindful Hunger and Fullness Scale:

1 - Extremely Hungry:

- Description: You're ravenous, and your body is signaling an urgent need for sustenance.

- Action: Start with a smaller portion to avoid overeating due to extreme hunger.

3 - Moderately Hungry:

- Description: You feel hungry but can wait a bit longer before eating.

- Action: Choose a balanced and satisfying meal to address your hunger.

5 - Neutral:

- Description: You're neither hungry nor full.

- Action: Recognize this neutral state as a baseline, and eat based on physical rather than emotional cues.

7 - Satisfied:

- Description: You're comfortably satisfied and content.

- Action: Pause and assess your fullness. Consider whether you genuinely need more food to feel satisfied.

9 - Very Full:

- Description: You feel overly full and may experience discomfort.

- Action: Stop eating and allow your body time to digest. Consider adjusting portion sizes in future meals.

10 - Uncomfortably Full:

- Description: You've surpassed a comfortable fullness level and may feel bloated or sluggish.

- Action: Reflect on the factors that led to overeating and use this awareness in future meals.

• Mindful Eating in Daily Life:

1. Snacking with Purpose:
   - Tip: Snack when you're genuinely hungry, choosing nutrient-dense options. Avoid snacking out of boredom or stress.

2. Intuitive Meal Timing:
   - Tip: Eat meals at times that align with your natural hunger patterns. Don't force yourself to eat on a strict schedule if you're not hungry.

3. Balanced Plate Approach:

- Tip: Create balanced meals that include a mix of proteins, carbohydrates, and fats. This helps satisfy nutritional needs and supports stable blood sugar levels.

4. Reflect on Emotional Eating:

- Tip: If you find yourself eating in response to emotions rather than hunger, explore alternative coping mechanisms such as journaling, walking, or talking to a friend.

Listening to your hunger and fullness is a transformative practice that fosters a healthier relationship with food. By tuning into these signals, you empower yourself to make mindful choices, nourishing your body with the awareness it deserves. Remember that every meal is an opportunity to honor your body's cues and cultivate a deeper connection with the act of eating.

✓ **Enjoying Meals at a Comfortable Pace**
• Savoring the Pleasures of Mindful Eating

In the fast-paced world we live in, the pace at which we consume our meals plays a crucial role in our overall well-being. Let's delve into the art of savoring each bite, understanding the benefits of a comfortable eating pace, and cultivating a more enjoyable dining experience.

• Understanding the Importance of Pace:

- Description: The pace at which you eat influences your body's ability to register fullness, aids in digestion, and contributes to a more mindful and pleasurable dining experience.

- Tip: Aim for a pace that allows you to savor the flavors and textures of your food.

• Key Principles of Enjoying Meals at a Comfortable Pace:

1. Mindful Chewing:

- Tip: Chew your food thoroughly. This not only aids in digestion but also allows you to fully appreciate the taste and texture of each bite.

2. Setting the Tone:

- Tip: Begin your meal with a moment of gratitude. Take a breath, and set a positive and mindful tone for the dining experience.

3. Put Down Utensils:

- Tip: Between bites, put down your utensils. This simple act encourages you to chew, savor, and be more aware of your eating pace.

4. Engaging the Senses:

- Tip: Engage your senses by appreciating the aroma, colors, and presentation of your food. This enhances the overall enjoyment of the meal.

5. Conscious Breathing:

- Tip: Take occasional pauses to breathe consciously. This helps you connect with your body's signals of hunger and fullness.

• Benefits of a Comfortable Eating Pace:

1. Improved Digestion:

- Description: Eating slowly allows your digestive system to function more efficiently, aiding in nutrient absorption and reducing the risk of digestive discomfort.

- Tip: Chew your food thoroughly to kickstart the digestion process in your mouth.

2. Enhanced Satisfaction:

- Description: A comfortable pace allows you to register fullness more accurately, preventing overeating and promoting a satisfying and balanced meal.

- Tip: Pause between bites to assess your level of fullness.

3. Mindful Eating:

- Description: Enjoying meals at a comfortable pace fosters mindfulness. It encourages you to be present, savor the moment, and appreciate the culinary experience.

- Tip: Focus on the flavors, textures, and overall experience of each bite.

4. Blood Sugar Regulation:

- Description: Eating slowly helps regulate blood sugar levels by allowing a more gradual release of glucose into the bloodstream.

- Tip: Pair a comfortable eating pace with balanced meals to support stable blood sugar levels.

• Practical Tips for Enjoying Meals:

1. Create a Relaxing Environment:

- Tip: Choose a calm and inviting space for your meals. Minimize distractions and create an atmosphere that allows you to focus on your food.

2. Set Realistic Time Windows:

- Tip: Allocate sufficient time for meals. Avoid rushing through them, especially during busy periods. Consider this time a valuable investment in your well-being.

3. Mindful Portioning:

- Tip: Serve yourself reasonable portions. This not only promotes mindful eating but also prevents the temptation to rush through a large meal.

4. Share and Engage:

- Tip: Share meals with family or friends. Engage in conversation to naturally slow down your eating pace and create a more enjoyable dining atmosphere.

5. Practice Gratitude:

- Tip:Before taking the first bite, express gratitude for the nourishment in front of you. This simple practice sets a positive tone for the meal.

Enjoying meals at a comfortable pace is a simple yet profound practice that enhances your connection with food and contributes to overall well-being. By savoring each bite, engaging your senses, and cultivating mindfulness, you not only promote optimal digestion and blood sugar regulation but also elevate the act of eating into a pleasurable and nourishing experience.

CHAPTER 7

REVAMPING RECIPES FOR HEALTH

*T*ransforming Flavor with Nourishing Choices

In the pursuit of a healthier lifestyle, revamping recipes becomes a delightful and empowering journey. Let's explore the principles of making mindful ingredient choices, preserving the essence of flavor, and transforming your favorite dishes into nourishing culinary delights.

• Understanding Recipe Revamping:

   - Description: Recipe revamping involves making conscious choices to enhance the nutritional profile of a dish without compromising on taste. It's an opportunity to explore wholesome ingredients and create meals that support your well-being.

   - Tip: Embrace the process with curiosity and an open mind.

• Key Principles of Recipe Revamping:

1. Ingredient Substitutions:

- Tip: Substitute refined grains with whole grains, replace saturated fats with healthier fats, and explore alternative sweeteners to reduce added sugars.

2. Boosting Nutrient Density:
- Tip: Choose ingredients that pack a nutritional punch. Incorporate colorful vegetables, lean proteins, and fiber-rich grains to enhance the overall nutrient content.

3. Balancing Flavors:
- Tip: Experiment with herbs, spices, and aromatics to add depth and complexity to your dishes. Balancing flavors ensures a satisfying and enjoyable eating experience.

4. Mindful Cooking Techniques:

- Tip: Opt for cooking methods that retain the nutritional value of ingredients. Explore methods like steaming, roasting, or sautéing with minimal oil.

5. Reducing Sodium and Processed Ingredients:

- Tip: Gradually decrease the use of processed and high-sodium ingredients. Utilize herbs, citrus, and other natural flavor enhancers to replace excess salt.

• Practical Tips for Recipe Revamping:

1. Whole Grains Makeover:

- Tip: Substitute refined grains with whole grains in recipes. Choose quinoa, brown rice, or whole wheat pasta to increase fiber and nutrient content.

2. Lean Protein Choices:

- Tip: Opt for lean protein sources such as skinless poultry, fish, tofu, or legumes. These choices contribute to muscle health and satiety.

3. Vibrant Veggie Infusion:

- Tip: Increase the vegetable content in recipes. Sneak in extra veggies into sauces, stews, and casseroles for added vitamins and minerals.

4. Healthy Fats Upgrade:

- Tip: Replace saturated fats with healthier fats like olive oil, avocado, or nuts. These fats support heart health and add a rich, satisfying flavor.

5. Mindful Sweeteners:

- Tip: Explore natural sweeteners like honey, maple syrup, or agave nectar as alternatives to refined sugars. These options add sweetness without the same impact on blood sugar.

6. Portion Control Awareness:
   - Tip: Be mindful of portion sizes. Enjoying smaller portions allows you to savor the flavors while maintaining a balance in your overall diet.

7. Homemade Flavor Boosters:
   - Tip: Create homemade sauces, dressings, and spice blends. This allows you to control ingredients, reducing the reliance on store-bought, often high-sugar options.

• Benefits of Recipe Revamping:

1. Enhanced Nutritional Profile:

   - Description: Revamping recipes increases the nutrient density of your meals, providing essential vitamins, minerals, and other beneficial compounds.

   - Tip: Prioritize ingredients that contribute to your overall health goals.

2. Blood Sugar Regulation:

   - Description: Choosing whole, unprocessed ingredients supports stable blood sugar levels. This is particularly beneficial for individuals managing diabetes or looking to prevent blood sugar spikes.

   - Tip: Integrate complex carbohydrates, lean proteins, and healthy fats into your revamped recipes.

3. Heart Health Support:

- Description: Opting for healthier fats and incorporating heart-friendly ingredients promotes cardiovascular well-being.

- Tip: Include omega-3 fatty acids from sources like fatty fish, flaxseeds, and walnuts.

Revamping recipes for health is an enjoyable and rewarding endeavor that allows you to nourish your body while relishing the pleasure of good food. By making mindful ingredient choices, balancing flavors, and exploring creative substitutions, you transform meals into vibrant and satisfying culinary experiences. Embrace the journey of culinary exploration, and savor the positive impact on your overall well-being.

✓ **Transforming Favorites into Diabetes-Friendly Versions**
• Nourishing Traditions with a Healthier Twist

In the journey of managing diabetes, transforming favorite dishes becomes an opportunity to embrace a diabetes-friendly lifestyle without compromising on taste. Let's delve into the principles of making mindful ingredient choices, balancing carbohydrates, and creating versions of beloved recipes that support stable blood sugar levels.

• Understanding Diabetes-Friendly Transformations:

- Description: Transforming favorites into diabetes-friendly versions involves making thoughtful adjustments to reduce refined carbohydrates, control portion sizes, and emphasize nutrient-dense ingredients.

- Tip: Approach this process as an exploration of nourishing alternatives rather than a restriction.

• Key Principles of Diabetes-Friendly Transformations:

1. Carbohydrate Awareness:

- Tip: Be mindful of carbohydrate content. Opt for whole, complex carbohydrates and balance them with proteins and healthy fats to slow down the impact on blood sugar.

2. Portion Control:
   - Tip: Manage portion sizes to avoid large spikes in blood sugar. Consider using smaller plates to naturally control serving sizes.

3. Fiber-Rich Ingredients:
   - Tip: Integrate fiber-rich foods such as vegetables, legumes, and whole grains. Fiber slows down the absorption of glucose, promoting stable blood sugar levels.

4. Healthy Cooking Techniques:
   - Tip: Choose cooking methods that retain the nutritional value of ingredients. Grilling, roasting, steaming,

and sautéing with minimal oil are diabetes-friendly options.

5. Sugar Substitutes:

  - Tip: Experiment with sugar substitutes like stevia, erythritol, or monk fruit in moderation. These alternatives add sweetness without causing spikes in blood sugar.

• Practical Tips for Diabetes-Friendly Transformations:

1. Whole Grains Makeover:

  - Tip: Replace refined grains with whole grains. Choose brown rice, quinoa, or whole wheat pasta to increase fiber and nutrients.

2. Lean Protein Choices:

- Tip: Opt for lean protein sources. Include skinless poultry, fish, tofu, and legumes to support blood sugar control and overall health.

3. Vegetable-Centric Adaptations:
- Tip: Increase the vegetable-to-carbohydrate ratio in dishes. Enhance flavors with colorful vegetables while reducing reliance on starches.

4. Mindful Sweeteners:
- Tip: Choose natural sweeteners in moderation. Experiment with alternatives like cinnamon or vanilla to add sweetness without excessive sugar.

5. Balanced Plate Approach:

- Tip: Create balanced meals that include a mix of carbohydrates, proteins, and healthy fats. This combination supports blood sugar stability.

6. Culinary Herb Magic:
- Tip: Elevate flavors with herbs and spices. Experiment with basil, thyme, garlic, or ginger to add depth without relying on excessive salt or sugar.

• Benefits of Diabetes-Friendly Transformations:

1. Blood Sugar Regulation:
- Description: Transforming favorites into diabetes-friendly versions supports stable blood sugar levels. Balanced

meals with controlled carbohydrates contribute to better glucose control.

- Tip: Monitor your blood sugar responses to different meals and adjust recipes accordingly.

2. Nutrient-Rich Choices:

- Description: Emphasizing nutrient-dense ingredients provides essential vitamins and minerals, supporting overall health and well-being.

- Tip: Choose ingredients that offer a variety of nutrients to enhance the nutritional value of your meals.

3. Sustainable Lifestyle:

- Description: Diabetes-friendly transformations contribute to a sustainable and enjoyable lifestyle. By creating versions of your favorite dishes that align with your health goals, you can maintain a positive relationship with food.

- Tip: Share these transformations with friends and family to foster a supportive and health-conscious environment.

Transforming favorites into diabetes-friendly versions is a creative and empowering process that allows you to continue enjoying the flavors you love while prioritizing your health. By making mindful choices, balancing nutrients, and exploring alternative ingredients, you transform traditional recipes into nourishing and diabetes-friendly delights. Embrace the journey of culinary exploration, and savor the positive impact on your well-being and blood sugar management.

✓ Cooking for Joyful Wellness
• Embracing Culinary Joy for Holistic Well-Being

In the realm of wellness, cooking becomes a powerful and joyful tool to nourish both body and soul. Let's delve into the principles of cooking for joyful wellness, celebrating the pleasures of creating delicious and wholesome meals that contribute to a balanced and fulfilling life.

• Understanding Joyful Wellness in Cooking:

- Description: Cooking for joyful wellness goes beyond the functional aspect of preparing meals. It involves cultivating a positive and mindful relationship with the culinary process, deriving pleasure from nourishing both the body and the spirit.

- Tip: Approach cooking as a form of self-care and a creative expression of well-being.

• Key Principles of Cooking for Joyful Wellness:

1. Mindful Preparation:

- Tip: Engage in the cooking process with mindfulness. Pay attention to each ingredient, savor the aromas, and appreciate the textures to enhance the overall experience.

2. Culinary Creativity:

- Tip: Embrace your creativity in the kitchen. Experiment with flavors, try new recipes, and adapt dishes to your personal taste preferences.

3. Positive Affirmation:

- Tip: Affirm the positive aspects of cooking. Acknowledge the joy that the process brings, and view it as a rewarding and nourishing activity for both body and soul.

4. Sharing the Culinary Journey:

- Tip: Share the cooking experience with loved ones. Cooking together fosters connection, creating a shared space for joy and well-being.

5. Celebration of Ingredients:
   - Tip: Celebrate the variety and freshness of ingredients. Choose seasonal and colorful produce to infuse vibrancy and nutritional richness into your meals.

• Practical Tips for Joyful Wellness in Cooking:

1. Music and Atmosphere:
   - Tip: Create a joyful cooking atmosphere with music that inspires and uplifts. Let the rhythm of your favorite tunes infuse energy into the culinary experience.

2. Gratitude Ritual:
   - Tip: Begin each cooking session with a moment of gratitude. Express

thanks for the ingredients, the ability to prepare a meal, and the joy that cooking brings.

3. Slow Cooking Mindset:
   - Tip: Embrace a slow cooking mindset. Allow yourself the luxury of time to enjoy the process, savoring each step from preparation to presentation.

4. Seasonal Delights:
   - Tip: Explore seasonal ingredients and recipes. Seasonal cooking not only provides fresh and flavorful options but also connects you with the natural rhythm of the culinary calendar.

5. Culinary Rituals:
   - Tip: Develop personal culinary rituals. Whether it's the way you chop

vegetables or the order in which you add ingredients, rituals can enhance the sense of joy and familiarity in cooking.

• Benefits of Cooking for Joyful Wellness:

1. Stress Reduction:
   - Description: Cooking with joy and mindfulness can be a powerful stress-relieving activity. The act of creating in the kitchen becomes a therapeutic and enjoyable experience.
   - Tip: Use cooking as a mindful activity to unwind and focus on the present moment.

2. Enhanced Flavor Perception:
   - Description: When approached with joy and positivity, cooking becomes an

opportunity to explore and appreciate flavors more deeply. Enhanced flavor perception adds to the overall enjoyment of meals.

- Tip: Take moments to taste and savor your creations during the cooking process.

3. Culinary Connection:

- Description: Cooking for joyful wellness fosters a connection between mind, body, and the culinary experience. It becomes a form of self-expression and an avenue for cultivating overall well-being.

- Tip: Share your joy of cooking with others, creating a sense of connection and community.

Cooking for joyful wellness is a transformative practice that elevates the act of preparing meals to a joyful and nourishing experience. By infusing positivity, mindfulness, and creativity into your culinary journey, you not only nourish your body but also cultivate a sense of joy and fulfillment that contributes to your overall well-being.

CHAPTER 8

CONFIDENT DINING OUT

*N*avigating Restaurant Menus with Health and Flavor in Mind

Dining out should be a delightful experience that aligns with your health goals. Let's delve into the principles of confident dining out, equipping you with the knowledge and strategies to make informed choices that balance both taste and well-being.

• Understanding Confident Dining Out:
   - Description: Confident dining out involves navigating restaurant menus with a balance of health-conscious

choices and culinary enjoyment. It's about making informed decisions that align with your nutritional preferences while savoring the dining experience.

- Tip: Approach dining out as an opportunity to explore diverse flavors and cuisines without compromising your well-being.

• Key Principles of Confident Dining Out:

1. Menu Exploration:

- Tip: Take the time to explore the menu thoroughly. Look for dishes that incorporate a variety of nutrients, including lean proteins, whole grains, and vibrant vegetables.

2. Portion Awareness:

- Tip: Be mindful of portion sizes. Consider sharing dishes or opting for smaller portions to enjoy a variety without overindulging.

3. Balance of Nutrients:

- Tip: Aim for a balanced meal that includes proteins, healthy fats, and carbohydrates. This combination supports satiety and provides a well-rounded nutritional profile.

4. Smart Beverage Choices:

- Tip: Choose beverages wisely. Opt for water, herbal teas, or beverages with minimal added sugars to stay hydrated without unnecessary calories.

5. Customization Requests:

- Tip: Don't hesitate to customize your order. Ask for substitutions or adjustments to meet your dietary preferences, such as choosing a side of vegetables instead of fries.

• Practical Tips for Confident Dining Out:

1. Pre-Viewing Menus:
   - Tip: If possible, review the menu online before arriving. This allows you to plan your choices in advance and avoid impulsive decisions.

2. Mindful Appetizer Choices:
   - Tip: Start with a mindful choice of appetizer, such as a salad or broth-based soup. This can help control appetite and contribute to overall nutritional intake.

3. Grilled and Steamed Options:

- Tip: Look for grilled or steamed options on the menu. These cooking methods often involve less added fat and preserve the natural flavors of ingredients.

4. Sauces on the Side:

- Tip: Ask for sauces and dressings on the side. This gives you control over the amount you use, preventing overconsumption of added sugars and fats.

5. Allergen Inquiries:

- Tip: If you have specific dietary concerns or allergies, don't hesitate to inquire about ingredients and preparation methods. Most restaurants are accommodating and willing to provide information.

• Benefits of Confident Dining Out:

1. Mindful Choices for Well-Being:
    - Description: Confident dining out allows you to make mindful choices that align with your health goals. It empowers you to enjoy restaurant meals without compromising your well-being.
    - Tip: Focus on the pleasure of savoring delicious and nourishing dishes.

2. Variety and Culinary Exploration:
    - Description: By navigating menus confidently, you open yourself to a variety of flavors and culinary experiences. Dining out becomes an

opportunity for exploration and enjoyment.

- Tip: Embrace the diversity of cuisines and dishes offered by different restaurants.

3. Social Enjoyment:

- Description: Confident dining out enhances the social aspect of sharing meals with friends and family. You can participate fully in the dining experience while maintaining your health-conscious choices.

- Tip: Share your preferences with dining companions, fostering a supportive and health-conscious environment.

Confident dining out is a skill that enhances your overall dining experience, allowing you to savor delicious meals while maintaining a health-conscious approach. By applying the principles of menu exploration, portion awareness, and balanced choices, you can navigate restaurant menus with confidence and enjoy the pleasures of dining out without compromise.

✓ **Strategies for Success at Restaurants**
• Navigating Restaurant Dining with Confidence and Health in Mind

Dining at restaurants can be both enjoyable and health-conscious. Let's delve into practical strategies that empower you to make informed choices, ensuring a successful and satisfying restaurant experience that aligns with your well-being.

• Understanding Strategies for Success:

- Description: Strategies for success at restaurants involve a combination of mindfulness, preparation, and informed decision-making. These strategies empower you to enjoy the dining experience while prioritizing health-conscious choices.

- Tip: Adopting these strategies turns restaurant dining into an opportunity for both culinary pleasure and well-being.

• Key Strategies for Success:

1. Research and Choose Wisely:

- Tip: Prior to dining out, research restaurant menus online. Choose establishments that offer a variety of health-conscious options, making it easier to align with your dietary preferences.

2. Portion Control Planning:
    - Tip: Plan for portion control by deciding in advance whether you'll share dishes, order appetizers as main courses, or request a to-go box at the beginning of the meal to control portion sizes.

3. Mindful Beverage Choices:
    - Tip: Opt for water, unsweetened tea, or sparkling water to accompany your meal. This helps hydrate without adding unnecessary calories or sugars.

4. Prefer Grilled or Steamed Options:

- Tip: Choose dishes that are grilled, steamed, or baked. These cooking methods often involve less added fat, preserving the natural flavors of the ingredients.

5. Customization and Substitutions:

- Tip: Don't hesitate to customize your order. Ask for substitutions or modifications to meet your dietary preferences, such as requesting a side of vegetables instead of fries.

6. Navigate the Menu Mindfully:

- Tip: Mindfully navigate the menu by scanning for keywords like grilled, roasted, or steamed. These terms often indicate healthier cooking methods.

7. Be Allergen-Aware:

   - Tip: If you have dietary restrictions or allergies, communicate them to your server. Most restaurants are accommodating and can provide information on allergens in their dishes.

8. Share and Savor:

   - Tip: Consider sharing dishes with dining companions. This allows you to enjoy a variety of flavors without overindulging in large portions.

• Practical Tips for Success:

1. Smart Pre-Meal Snacking:

   - Tip: Have a small, nutritious snack before heading to the restaurant to curb excessive hunger and prevent impulsive, less health-conscious choices.

2. Pause Before Ordering:

- Tip: Take a moment to review the menu thoroughly before placing your order. This brief pause allows for thoughtful decision-making.

3. Mindful Eating Practices:

- Tip: Practice mindful eating by chewing slowly, savoring each bite, and paying attention to feelings of fullness. This enhances the overall dining experience.

4. Balanced Plate Approach:

- Tip: Strive for a balanced plate by including a mix of lean proteins, whole grains, and colorful vegetables. This ensures a well-rounded and satisfying meal.

5. Enjoy Desserts Mindfully:
    - Tip: If you choose to indulge in dessert, share it with others or ask for a smaller portion. Savor the sweetness mindfully.

• Benefits of Successful Dining Strategies:

1. Health-Conscious Choices:
    - Description: Implementing these strategies empowers you to make health-conscious choices at restaurants, supporting your overall well-being.
    - Tip: Focus on the satisfaction of making choices that align with your health goals.

2. Enhanced Dining Enjoyment:

    - Description: Successful dining strategies enhance the overall enjoyment of the dining experience. You can savor the flavors, connect with others, and appreciate the culinary journey.

   - Tip: Embrace the pleasure of dining out while making choices that contribute to your well-being.

3. Confident and Informed Decisions:

    - Description: These strategies instill confidence and ensure that you make informed decisions when faced with restaurant menus. You can navigate options with clarity and purpose.

- Tip: Trust your ability to make choices that align with your health-conscious goals.

Strategies for success at restaurants empower you to navigate dining options with confidence and well-being in mind. By incorporating mindfulness, planning, and informed decision-making, you can transform restaurant dining into a successful and satisfying experience that supports your health-conscious lifestyle.

✓ **Navigating Social Eating with Ease**

• Balancing Social Enjoyment and Well-Being

Social eating is a significant part of life's celebrations and gatherings. Let's delve into strategies that empower you to navigate social occasions with ease, striking a balance between enjoying the company of others and maintaining your health-conscious choices.

• Understanding Social Eating with Ease:

- Description: Navigating social eating with ease involves approaching gatherings and events with a balanced mindset—embracing the joy of social connections while making health-conscious choices.

- Tip: View social occasions as opportunities to enjoy both the company of others and nourishing, mindful food choices.

• Key Strategies for Navigating Social Eating:

1. Pre-Event Preparation:
    - Tip: Before attending an event, consider eating a balanced snack or light meal. This helps curb excessive hunger, making it easier to make mindful choices during the event.

2. Survey the Spread Mindfully:
    - Tip: Take a moment to survey the food offerings at social gatherings. Identify healthier options and plan your plate accordingly.

3. Moderation and Variety:
    - Tip: Practice moderation by enjoying a variety of dishes in smaller

portions. This allows you to savor flavors without overindulging.

4. Hydration Habits:

- Tip: Stay hydrated with water or other low-calorie beverages. This not only supports overall well-being but also helps manage appetite.

5. Prioritize Social Connections:

- Tip: Focus on the social aspects of gatherings rather than solely on the food. Engage in conversations, connect with others, and make the event about shared experiences.

• Practical Tips for Navigating Social Eating:

1. Mindful Plate Composition:

- Tip: Construct your plate mindfully by including a balance of proteins, vegetables, and whole grains. This ensures a variety of nutrients and flavors.

2. Plan Indulgences Mindfully:

- Tip: If there are indulgent treats at the event, plan to enjoy them mindfully. Savor each bite and focus on the pleasure of the experience.

3. Strategic Seating Choices:

- Tip: Choose seating arrangements strategically. Position yourself away from the buffet or snack table to reduce mindless grazing.

4. Practice Saying No Gracefully:

- Tip: Learn to decline politely when offered food that doesn't align with your health goals. You can express gratitude and share that you're satisfied with what you have.

5. Bring a Healthy Dish:

- Tip: If appropriate, bring a healthy dish to share. This ensures there's an option you feel comfortable including in your meal.

• Benefits of Navigating Social Eating with Ease:

1. Balanced Well-Being:

- Description: Navigating social eating with ease contributes to a balanced sense of well-being. You can enjoy social occasions without feeling restricted or compromising your health goals.

- Tip: Embrace the holistic enjoyment of both social connections and mindful food choices.

2. Positive Relationship with Food:

- Description: By making health-conscious choices at social events, you foster a positive relationship with food. It becomes a source of pleasure rather than stress.

- Tip: Celebrate the joy of sharing meals with others while maintaining your health-conscious mindset.

3. Sustainable Social Habits:

- Description: These strategies cultivate sustainable social habits. You can consistently engage in gatherings, celebrations, and events without feeling overwhelmed or disconnected from your health goals.

- Tip: Share your approach with friends and family to create a supportive and health-conscious social environment.

Navigating social eating with ease is an empowering skill that allows you to engage in social occasions while maintaining a health-conscious approach to food. By implementing practical strategies and prioritizing the joy of social connections, you can strike a harmonious balance that supports both well-being and enjoyment.

CHAPTER 9

EXERCISE AND NUTRITION WORKING TOGETHER

*I*n the bustling tapestry of well-being, the synergy between exercise and nutrition forms a dynamic duo—an alliance that extends beyond physical appearance to the very core of our vitality. This chapter delves into the intricate dance of these two pillars, unraveling the secrets of how they collaborate for optimal health.

• Understanding the Interconnected Web:

At its essence, the interplay between exercise and nutrition is a web of intricate connections. To comprehend this dynamic relationship, we must journey into the realms of metabolism, energy expenditure, and the symbiotic exchange that occurs within our bodies.

• Metabolism Unveiled:

Metabolism, the body's biochemical process of converting food into energy, takes center stage. Exercise becomes the catalyst that propels metabolism into a state of heightened efficiency. As we move, our muscles demand energy, and the metabolic engine revs up, burning calories not only during the activity but also in the post-exercise recovery period.

• Nutrient Fuel for the Engine:

Just as a car requires quality fuel for optimal performance, our bodies demand nutrient-rich sustenance. Carbohydrates emerge as the primary energy source, providing the quick fuel needed for high-intensity exercise. Proteins step onto the stage, aiding in muscle repair and growth, while fats contribute to sustained energy during more prolonged activities.

• Fueling Your Workouts:

Understanding that not all workouts are created equal, the concept of fueling becomes paramount. Whether engaging in cardio, strength training, or a combination of both, the body's fuel requirements vary.

• Pre-Workout Nutrition:

Before embarking on the exercise journey, pre-workout nutrition sets the stage. A balance of carbohydrates and proteins becomes the prelude, offering readily available energy and priming the muscles for the impending activity. Timing matters, and the goal is to consume a well-rounded meal or snack about 1–3 hours before the workout.

• During-Workout Hydration:

Amidst the exertion, hydration emerges as a steadfast companion. Water, often underestimated in its significance, plays a crucial role in maintaining performance. For more prolonged activities, the inclusion of electrolytes helps replenish what is lost through sweat, ensuring the body stays hydrated and functional.

• Post-Workout Recovery:

As the workout concludes, the spotlight shifts to post-workout recovery. The body craves a blend of protein and carbohydrates to repair muscles, replenish glycogen stores, and optimize recovery. This period becomes a golden opportunity to nurture the body, aiding its adaptation and growth.

• Moving Toward Balance:

Balance becomes the overarching theme in the interplay between exercise and nutrition. Striking the right balance ensures that the body receives the nourishment it requires to support physical activity without unnecessary strain.

• Adapting to Individual Needs:

Recognizing that each person's journey is unique, adaptation becomes a guiding principle. Individual needs, goals, and preferences shape the balance between exercise and nutrition. Whether aiming for weight loss, muscle gain, or simply overall health, customization is the key.

• Caloric Balance and Beyond:

Beyond the simplistic notion of caloric balance, the quality of calories assumes paramount importance. Nutrient-dense foods not only contribute to overall health but also offer the sustained energy required for consistent exercise.

• Fueling the Flames of Well-Being:

The harmonious interplay between exercise and nutrition extends its influence far beyond physical fitness. Mental health, immune function, and even sleep quality find themselves under the benevolent umbrella of this symbiotic relationship.

• Mental Health Resonance:

Exercise's ability to stimulate the release of endorphins, coupled with proper nutrition supporting brain function, creates a powerful alliance for mental health. The mood-enhancing effects of physical activity intertwine with the cognitive benefits of a well-nourished brain.

• Immune System Support:

Nutrition emerges as a silent guardian of the immune system. Adequate intake of vitamins and minerals fortifies the body's defenses, while regular exercise contributes to immune system regulation. The harmonious duo stands as a fortress against illness and supports overall well-being.

• The Sleep Connection:

As the day unfolds, the quality of sleep becomes a reflection of the harmony between exercise and nutrition. Physical activity promotes restorative sleep, while proper nutrition provides the nutrients necessary for the body's nighttime repair processes.

• Practical Tips for Integration:

Embarking on a journey toward optimal health requires practical strategies. Incorporating exercise and nutrition into daily life becomes not just a goal but a tangible reality.

• Creating Balanced Meals:

Building meals that encompass a variety of nutrients ensures the body receives a comprehensive spectrum of essential elements. Colorful fruits and vegetables, lean proteins, whole grains, and healthy fats become the palette for crafting nutritionally rich meals.

• Adapting to Exercise Preferences:

Acknowledging that exercise is not one-size-fits-all, individuals are encouraged to discover activities they enjoy. From brisk walks to weightlifting, the key lies in finding joy in movement, ensuring sustained engagement over the long term.

• Mindful Eating and Exercise:

The art of mindful eating aligns seamlessly with the principles of exercise and nutrition. Paying attention to hunger and fullness cues, savoring flavors, and cultivating a mindful approach to both nourishment and movement weave a tapestry of holistic well-being.

• Fostering a Lifelong Connection:

In concluding our exploration of exercise and nutrition, the emphasis shifts toward fostering a lifelong connection. The transient nature of fad diets and extreme workout regimens fades in comparison to the enduring impact of sustainable habits.

• Sustainability Over Extremes:

Sustainable habits that can be integrated into daily life take precedence over extreme approaches. The goal is not a sprint but a marathon—a journey where exercise and nutrition become steadfast companions in the tapestry of well-being.

• Celebrating Progress, Not Perfection:

Recognizing that perfection is an elusive ideal, the focus shifts to celebrating progress. Small, consistent steps toward integrating positive habits become the milestones of a journey that spans a lifetime.

• A Holistic Symphony of Wellness:

In the grand symphony of well-being, exercise and nutrition emerge not as isolated notes but as harmonious chords, creating a melody that reverberates through the dimensions of our physical, mental, and emotional realms.

✓ **Moving Toward Balance**
• Embracing Holistic Well-Being for a Balanced Life

Moving toward balance involves aligning different facets of life to achieve overall well-being. This chapter delves into the key elements of balance, emphasizing the importance of harmony in nutrition, exercise, mental well-being, and lifestyle choices.

• Understanding the Pursuit of Balance:

   - Description: Moving toward balance is a journey of harmonizing different aspects of life. It involves cultivating a holistic approach that embraces nutrition, exercise, stress management, and self-care to achieve a state of overall well-being.

   - Tip: Approach balance as an ongoing process rather than a destination, allowing for continuous growth and adaptation.

• Key Elements of Moving Toward Balance:

1. Mindful Nutrition:

   - Tip: Practice mindful eating by savoring flavors, paying attention to hunger and fullness cues, and choosing nourishing foods that support your overall health.

2. Adaptable Exercise Routine:

   - Tip: Create an exercise routine that aligns with your preferences and goals. Aim for a mix of cardiovascular, strength, and flexibility exercises to support overall fitness.

3. Stress Management Strategies:

   - Tip: Incorporate stress management techniques such as meditation, deep breathing, or mindfulness into your daily routine. These practices contribute to mental well-being and balance.

4. Adequate Rest and Recovery:
   - Tip: Prioritize sufficient sleep and recovery. Quality rest is essential for physical and mental rejuvenation, supporting overall balance in your life.

• Practical Integration of Balance:

1. Holistic Self-Care:
   - Tip: Embrace holistic self-care practices. This may include activities such as spending time in nature, pursuing hobbies, or engaging in activities that bring joy and relaxation.

2. Lifestyle Adaptations:

- Tip: Assess your lifestyle and make adaptations that promote balance. This may involve setting boundaries, delegating tasks, or simplifying commitments to create more space for well-being.

3. Continuous Learning and Growth:
   - Tip: Foster a mindset of continuous learning and growth. Seek opportunities for personal and professional development that align with your values and contribute to a sense of fulfillment.

• Benefits of Moving Toward Balance:

1. Enhanced Well-Being:
   - Description: Moving toward balance enhances overall well-being, encompassing physical, mental, and

emotional aspects of health. It creates a foundation for a fulfilling and purpose-driven life.

- Tip: Celebrate the small victories and positive changes along your journey toward balance.

2. Resilience in Life Challenges:

- Description: A balanced lifestyle fosters resilience in the face of life's challenges. By nurturing physical and mental well-being, you develop the capacity to navigate stress and uncertainty with greater ease.

- Tip: Cultivate resilience through self-compassion and the ability to adapt to changing circumstances.

3. Sustainable Healthy Habits:

- Description: The pursuit of balance supports the development of sustainable healthy habits. Rather than relying on short-term fixes, you establish a foundation for long-term well-being.

- Tip: Focus on creating habits that align with your values and contribute positively to your life.

Moving toward balance is a dynamic and personal journey that involves integrating various elements of well-being. By embracing mindful nutrition, adaptable exercise routines, stress management, and holistic self-care, you create a foundation for a balanced and fulfilling life. Remember, balance is not a perfect state but an ongoing process of growth and self-discovery.

✓ Fueling Your Workouts for Optimal Health

• Nourishing Your Body for Peak Performance

Fueling your workouts is a key component of achieving optimal health. This chapter delves into the importance of providing your body with the right nutrients before, during, and after exercise, ensuring that you can perform at your best and support your overall well-being.

• Understanding Optimal Workout Fueling:

- Description: Optimal workout fueling involves providing your body with the necessary nutrients to support energy levels, enhance performance, and aid recovery. It's a strategic approach to nourishing your body for peak physical activity and overall health.

- Tip: Tailor your nutritional strategy based on the type, intensity, and duration of your workouts.

• Key Elements of Optimal Workout Fueling:

1. Pre-Workout Nutrition:

- Tip: Consume a balanced meal or snack containing carbohydrates, proteins, and a small amount of healthy fats before exercising. This provides a readily available energy source for your workout.

2. Hydration Before and During:

   - Tip: Ensure proper hydration before and during your workout. Dehydration can negatively impact performance and hinder the body's ability to regulate temperature.

3. Intra-Workout Nutrition (for Longer Sessions):

   - Tip: For longer or more intense workouts, consider incorporating intra-workout nutrition. This may involve consuming carbohydrates and electrolytes to sustain energy levels.

4. Post-Workout Refueling:

   - Tip: Prioritize a post-workout meal or snack rich in protein and carbohydrates. This aids in muscle recovery, replenishes glycogen stores, and supports overall recovery.

• Practical Strategies for Optimal Workout Fueling:

1. Customized Nutrition Plans:
   - Tip: Tailor your nutrition plans to your individual needs, considering factors such as workout intensity, duration, and personal preferences. Experiment to find what works best for you.

2. Timing and Quantity Considerations:
   - Tip: Pay attention to the timing and quantity of your pre-workout meal or snack. Optimal fueling depends on factors such as when you exercise and

your body's individual response to different foods.

3. Balanced Macronutrient Intake:

- Tip: Aim for a balance of carbohydrates, proteins, and fats in your overall diet. Each macronutrient plays a role in supporting different aspects of exercise performance and recovery.

4. Supplementation When Necessary:

- Tip: Consider supplementation, if needed. Certain situations, such as intense training or specific dietary restrictions, may benefit from supplements like protein powders, electrolyte replacements, or energy gels.

Benefits of Optimal Workout Fueling:

1. Enhanced Exercise Performance:

- Description: Optimal workout fueling enhances exercise performance by providing the necessary energy and nutrients. This translates to improved endurance, strength, and overall physical capabilities.

- Tip: Experiment with different fueling strategies to find what positively impacts your performance.

2. Efficient Recovery:

- Description: Proper nutrition post-workout contributes to efficient recovery. It aids in muscle repair, reduces muscle soreness, and prepares your body for subsequent workouts.

- Tip: Prioritize post-workout refueling to optimize recovery and support long-term training goals.

3. Sustained Energy Levels:

- Description: Consistent, balanced fueling supports sustained energy levels throughout your workouts. This ensures that you can perform at your best and derive maximum benefits from your exercise routine.

- Tip: Listen to your body's signals and adjust your fueling strategy based on your energy needs.

Fueling your workouts for optimal health is a fundamental aspect of a well-rounded approach to physical activity. By strategically providing your body with the right nutrients, you not only enhance exercise performance but also contribute to overall well-being. Experiment with different fueling strategies, stay attuned to your body's responses, and make adjustments as needed to support your fitness goals and long-term health.

CHAPTER 10

BALANCING STRESS, SLEEP, AND BLOOD SUGAR

*T*he Interplay for Holistic Health

Balancing stress, sleep, and blood sugar is a dynamic interplay that significantly influences your overall health. This chapter delves into the intricate connections between these elements and provides insights into fostering a harmonious equilibrium for optimal well-being.

• Understanding the Interconnected Trio:

- Description: The delicate balance between stress, sleep, and blood sugar is integral to holistic health. Stress can impact sleep quality and disrupt blood sugar regulation, while adequate sleep and mindful stress management contribute to stable blood sugar levels.

- Tip: Approach these elements as interrelated components of a comprehensive well-being strategy.

• Key Elements of Balancing Stress, Sleep, and Blood Sugar:

1. Stress Management Techniques:

- Tip: Incorporate stress management techniques into your daily routine. Practices such as mindfulness, deep breathing, and physical activity can help mitigate the impact of stress on your body.

2. Prioritizing Quality Sleep:

- Tip: Prioritize quality sleep by establishing consistent sleep patterns, creating a conducive sleep environment, and practicing relaxation techniques before bedtime.

3. Mindful Blood Sugar Management:

- Tip: Adopt mindful blood sugar management by incorporating balanced meals, regular physical activity, and monitoring carbohydrate intake. This supports stable blood sugar levels throughout the day.

4. Holistic Lifestyle Choices:

- Tip: Make holistic lifestyle choices that promote overall well-being. This includes maintaining a healthy diet, engaging in regular exercise, and fostering positive social connections.

• Practical Strategies for Balance:

1. Daily Stress-Reducing Habits:

   - Tip: Cultivate daily habits that reduce stress, such as brief breaks for deep breathing, short walks, or moments of mindfulness. Consistent stress reduction contributes to long-term well-being.

2. Sleep Hygiene Practices:

   - Tip: Practice good sleep hygiene by creating a dark, quiet, and comfortable sleep environment. Limit screen time before bed and establish a consistent sleep schedule to support restful sleep.

3. Balanced Nutrition Choices:

   - Tip: Make balanced nutrition choices by incorporating a variety of nutrient-dense foods. Focus on whole grains, lean proteins, and colorful vegetables to support stable blood sugar levels.

4. Regular Physical Activity:
   - Tip: Engage in regular physical activity, as it not only supports overall health but also contributes to stress reduction and improved sleep quality.

• Benefits of Balance Across Stress, Sleep, and Blood Sugar:

1. Enhanced Emotional Well-Being:
   - Description: Balancing stress, sleep, and blood sugar enhances emotional well-being. By managing stress, prioritizing quality sleep, and stabilizing blood sugar levels, you foster a positive and resilient mindset.

- Tip: Cultivate emotional resilience through a holistic approach to well-being.

2. Optimal Physical Health:

- Description: The interplay between stress, sleep, and blood sugar contributes to optimal physical health. This includes improved immune function, better metabolism, and a reduced risk of chronic health conditions.

- Tip: View these elements as interconnected pillars supporting your overall physical well-being.

3. Sustainable Lifestyle Habits:

- Description: Achieving balance in stress, sleep, and blood sugar fosters sustainable lifestyle habits. Consistency in positive choices leads to long-term well-being and resilience in the face of life's challenges.

- Tip: Embrace these habits as a foundation for a healthy and fulfilling life.

Balancing stress, sleep, and blood sugar is a dynamic and interconnected process that significantly influences your overall health. By incorporating stress management techniques, prioritizing quality sleep, and adopting mindful blood sugar management, you create a foundation for holistic well-being.

✓ How Lifestyle Affects Diabetes

• The Power of Lifestyle Choices in Diabetes Prevention and Management

Understanding the intricate relationship between lifestyle choices and diabetes is key to effective prevention and management. This chapter explores how various aspects of lifestyle, including diet, physical activity, stress management, and sleep, can influence the development and progression of diabetes.

Introduction:

- Description: Lifestyle choices have a profound impact on diabetes, influencing both its onset and management. By making informed decisions related to nutrition, exercise, stress, and sleep, individuals can play an active role in preventing and managing diabetes.

- Tip: View lifestyle modifications as powerful tools for enhancing overall health and well-being.

• Key Aspects of Lifestyle and Diabetes:

1. Nutrition and Dietary Choices:
   - Tip: Adopting a balanced and mindful approach to nutrition is crucial. Focus on whole, nutrient-dense foods, control portion sizes, and be mindful of carbohydrate intake to help manage blood sugar levels effectively.

2. Regular Physical Activity:
   - Tip: Engage in regular physical activity to enhance insulin sensitivity, control weight, and promote overall cardiovascular health. Both aerobic

exercises and strength training play integral roles in diabetes prevention and management.

3. Stress Management Techniques:

- Tip: Chronic stress can impact blood sugar levels. Incorporate stress management techniques such as meditation, deep breathing, or yoga to mitigate stress and promote emotional well-being.

4. Quality Sleep Habits:

- Tip: Prioritize quality sleep by maintaining consistent sleep patterns and creating a conducive sleep environment. Poor sleep can affect insulin sensitivity and contribute to diabetes risk.

• Practical Strategies for Diabetes Prevention and Management:

1. Personalized Nutrition Plans:
   - Tip: Work with healthcare professionals to develop personalized nutrition plans that consider your dietary preferences, lifestyle, and diabetes management goals.

2. Tailored Exercise Routines:
   - Tip: Consult with fitness experts to create tailored exercise routines that align with your fitness level and diabetes management needs. Both aerobic and resistance exercises can be adapted to individual preferences.

3. Mindfulness and Relaxation Practices:

- Tip: Integrate mindfulness and relaxation practices into your daily routine. This not only contributes to stress reduction but also positively influences blood sugar control.

4. Consistent Blood Sugar Monitoring:

- Tip: For individuals with diabetes, consistent blood sugar monitoring is crucial. This information guides lifestyle adjustments and helps maintain optimal blood sugar levels.

• Benefits of Lifestyle Modifications for Diabetes:

1. Improved Blood Sugar Control:

- Description: Lifestyle modifications contribute to improved blood sugar control, reducing the risk of complications associated with diabetes. Consistent healthy choices positively impact glycemic levels.

- Tip: Regularly monitor blood sugar levels and observe how lifestyle changes influence your overall well-being.

2. Weight Management and Cardiovascular Health:

- Description: Lifestyle choices play a pivotal role in weight management and cardiovascular health. Maintaining a healthy weight and promoting cardiovascular fitness are integral aspects of diabetes prevention and management.

- Tip: Embrace a holistic approach that benefits both diabetes control and overall cardiovascular well-being.

3. Enhanced Quality of Life:

- Description: Lifestyle modifications enhance the overall quality of life for individuals with diabetes. By making informed choices, individuals can lead fulfilling, active lives while effectively managing their condition.

- Tip: Celebrate the positive changes and improvements in well-being as a result of lifestyle modifications.

Understanding how lifestyle choices affect diabetes empowers individuals to take an active role in their health. By embracing personalized nutrition plans, tailored exercise routines, stress management techniques, and consistent blood sugar monitoring, individuals can navigate the journey of diabetes prevention and management with confidence. Remember, every positive lifestyle choice contributes to a healthier, more vibrant life.

✓ Simple Approaches for Overall Wellbeing

• Everyday Practices for a Healthier and Happier Life

Fostering overall well-being doesn't always require complex changes. This chapter highlights simple and practical approaches that individuals can integrate into their daily routines to promote physical health, mental clarity, and emotional balance.

• Introduction:

- Description: Overall well-being is achievable through small, consistent actions integrated into daily life. These simple approaches encompass various aspects, including nutrition, physical activity, mindfulness, and connection, contributing to a healthier and happier life.

- Tip: Embrace simplicity and gradual progress on the journey toward overall well-being.

• Key Elements of Simple Approaches:

1. Nutrition Conscious Choices:

- Tip: Make nutrition-conscious choices by incorporating more whole, plant-based foods into your diet. Gradually reduce processed food intake and focus on mindful eating to savor flavors and promote digestion.

2. Move Throughout the Day:

- Tip: Incorporate movement into your daily routine. This can include short walks, stretching breaks, or simple exercises at home. Consistent movement contributes to physical health and mental clarity.

3. Mindful Moments:

- Tip: Integrate mindful moments into your day. Take a few minutes to practice deep breathing, observe your surroundings, or engage in brief meditation. These moments foster mental clarity and emotional balance.

4. Hydration Habits:

- Tip: Stay hydrated throughout the day by making water your primary beverage. Hydration supports various bodily functions and contributes to overall well-being.

Practical Strategies for Everyday Well-Being:

1. Create a Balanced Plate:
   - Tip: Aim for a balanced plate by including a variety of colorful vegetables, lean proteins, and whole grains. This ensures a diverse range of nutrients to support overall health.

2. Breaks for Movement:
   - Tip: Take short breaks for movement during the day. Whether it's a brisk walk, stretching exercises, or a quick

dance session, incorporating movement enhances physical well-being and mental focus.

3. Mindful Eating Practices:
    - Tip: Practice mindful eating by savoring each bite, paying attention to hunger and fullness cues, and minimizing distractions during meals. This approach enhances digestion and the overall dining experience.

4. Daily Hygiene of Mindfulness:
    - Tip: Cultivate a daily hygiene of mindfulness by incorporating brief moments of awareness into your routine. This can be as simple as taking a few mindful breaths before starting a task or appreciating a moment of stillness.

• Benefits of Simple Approaches for Well-Being:

1. Sustainable Lifestyle Habits:
   - Description: Simple approaches contribute to the development of sustainable lifestyle habits. These habits become ingrained in daily life, promoting long-term physical and mental well-being.
   - Tip: Focus on gradual progress and consistency rather than aiming for perfection.

2. Enhanced Energy and Vitality:
   - Description: Embracing simple approaches enhances overall energy levels and vitality. Making conscious choices in nutrition, movement, and

mindfulness fosters a sense of well-being and vigor.

- Tip: Observe how these simple changes positively impact your daily energy levels.

3. Improved Mood and Emotional Balance:

- Description: Incorporating mindful moments and movement into daily life contributes to improved mood and emotional balance. These practices provide a space for stress reduction and increased emotional resilience.

- Tip: Notice the positive shifts in your emotional well-being as you integrate these simple approaches.

Overall well-being is a journey made up of simple, everyday choices. By creating a balanced plate, incorporating movement, practicing mindfulness, and staying hydrated, individuals can cultivate a lifestyle that supports physical health, mental clarity, and emotional balance. Embrace these simple approaches as foundational elements on your path to a healthier and happier life.

CONCLUSION

In the tapestry of our exploration, each chapter has been a note in the symphony of well-being. From the initial endeavor of decoding carbs and understanding the intricate dance with diabetes to the nuanced exploration of balanced living and mindful choices, this journey has unfolded as a melody of transformation and self-discovery.

• A Journey of Unveiling:

Our venture began with the intention to unravel the mysteries of carbs and diabetes. As we progressed through the chapters, the narrative evolved into a profound exploration of not only managing diabetes but also fostering a holistic sense of well-being.

• Decoding the Complexity:

Delving into the fundamentals of why carbs matter, we traversed deeper into the basics, appreciating the significance of a balanced diet. The journey embraced the establishment of personal diabetes plans, laying resilient foundations adaptable to individual lifestyles.

• Nourishment Beyond the Cart:

Smart grocery shopping ceased to be a mundane task, becoming a conscious choice. Tips for a healthy cart and the skill of reading labels like a pro became tools of empowerment, shaping our nutritional journey.

• Crafting Culinary Symphony:

The realm of meal planning became a canvas for creativity. Crafting diabetes-friendly menus and embracing the convenience of batch cooking transformed mealtime into a celebration of health and joy.

• A Palette of Possibilities:

Exploring delicious carb alternatives, we not only found substitutes but uncovered a palette of possibilities. Tasty substitutes and the addition of excitement to our plates highlighted the joy that can be found in diverse and health-conscious culinary choices.

• Mindful Nourishment:

Eating mindfully emerged as a cornerstone, transforming meals into moments of connection with our bodies. Listening to hunger and fullness cues and enjoying meals at a comfortable pace brought mindfulness to the forefront of our dining experience.

• Culinary Alchemy:

Revamping recipes for health became a form of culinary alchemy. Transforming favorites into diabetes-friendly versions and cooking for joyful wellness illustrated the potential for nourishing our bodies without compromising on taste.

• Empowered Dining:

Confident dining out became an art of empowerment. Strategies for success at restaurants and navigating social eating with ease illuminated the possibility of maintaining health-conscious choices in various social settings.

• The Synergy of Movement and Nutrition:

The interplay between exercise and nutrition became a dynamic force in our pursuit of balance. Moving toward equilibrium and fueling our workouts for optimal health showcased the synergy between physical activity and well-being.

• A Harmonious Trio:

The grand finale explored the delicate equilibrium of stress, sleep, and blood sugar. Understanding how lifestyle affects diabetes, we embraced simple approaches, fostering a holistic well-being that extends beyond individual components.

• The Grand Finale:

As we conclude this symphony of well-being, let these words echo the sentiment of a journey well-traveled. May the melodies of balance, mindfulness, and intentional living resonate in every choice, creating a cadence of joy, health, and fulfillment.